Working Relationships

Practical Theology Series

This new series brings together accessible texts that combine in-depth consideration of theory with suggestions for caring practice. Drawing on the latest research and experience in a range of practice settings, these are informative and thought-provoking resources for practical theologians and practitioners working in health and social care.

Working Relationships

Spirituality in Human Service and Organisational Life

Neil Pembroke

Jessica Kingsley Publishers
London and New York

First published in the United Kingdom in 2004
by Jessica Kingsley Publishers Ltd
116 Pentonville Road
London N1 9JB, England
and
29 West 35th Street, 10th fl.
New York, NY 10001-2299, USA

www.jkp.com

Copyright © Neil Pembroke 2004

Library of Congress Cataloging in Publication Data
Pembroke, Neil.
Working relationships : spirituality in human service and organisational life / Neil Pembroke.
    p. cm. -- (Practical theology series)
Includes bibliographical references (p.   ) and index.
  ISBN 1-84310-252-8 (pbk.)
  1. Social service--Religious aspects. 2. Social service. I. Title. II. Series.
  HV530.P34 2004
  261.8'32--dc22
                                            2003026445

British Library Cataloguing in Publication Data
A CIP catalogue record for this book is available from the British Library

ISBN 1 84310 252 8

Printed and Bound in Great Britain by
Athenaeum Press, Gateshead, Tyne and Wear

For my wife, Janelle. My best friend.

Acknowledgements

There are some friends and colleagues who have given generously of their time and talents in making this a better book than it would otherwise have been. I deeply appreciate their contributions. Rev. Professor Han Spykerboer, formerly of Trinity Theological College, read an early version and made a number of very helpful comments. My wife, Janelle, has been a supportive and insightful conversation partner and has supplied me with some very useful midwifery articles. Finally, I would like to express my gratitude to Professor John Swinton, editor of the series, and to Ms Amy Lankester-Owen, Editorial Director at Jessica Kingsley Publishers, for their interest and affirmation. It really has been a joy working with them on this project.

Contents

Introduction

In this book, I provide a theological and ethical interpretation of relationships in human service acts and in the organisational life supporting those acts. I am interested in what it is that humanises or spiritualises working relationships in the sphere of human service. I should comment at the outset on my use of the term 'human service' and on my selection of professions. The term is used to refer to four professions, namely counselling and psychotherapy, teaching, nursing, and midwifery. These professionals have their own particular terms they commonly use to describe the service they provide (such as mental health services, education and health care). They will perhaps find the reference to their work as 'human service' slightly unusual. In fact, it is more commonly used with reference to various forms of social work. I am using 'human service' as a catch-all designator simply because the four professions I will be attending to do in fact service human beings. Some have also used the term 'personal service professions' as a generic term. 'Personal service' will also be used on occasion.

In explaining my terminology, I refer to the social work profession. This could also have been included in my treatment. The work of medical practitioners is another candidate; the same is true of physiotherapy, occupational therapy and the other allied health services. My aim, however, is not to be as comprehensive as possible, but rather to establish general principles and to illustrate them through references to a representative sample of human service professions.

It is perhaps important to say a little at the outset about my background and the context for my reflections on this issue. My doctoral research was in the area of Christian pastoral care. Influential in the way I do my pastoral theology is the contention of Don Browning and others that we need to broaden the scope of our concern in pastoral care. In his influential book *The Moral Context of Pastoral Care*, Browning (1976, p.20) observed that, historically, pastoral care has had two principal functions. The first has been to form members in the normative vision of the Christian church. The second, to support persons as they attempt to cope with various developmental, emotional and existential crises. Browning argued that pastoral theologians, pastors and laypersons all need to give much more attention to the first function. For him, the church should be a place where lively and wide-ranging moral discourse is a central feature (Browning 1976, p.91). We need, Browning contended, to be constantly developing and refining our theologies of important life issues such as marriage, sexuality, divorce, ageing and work.

Since Browning's book came out, a number of pastoral theologians have joined with him in arguing for attention to a wider range of concerns and issues. Such an approach is necessary to develop a comprehensive understanding of what constitutes physical, emotional and spiritual well-being. Personal well-being cannot be interpreted solely in terms of intrapsychic and interpersonal dynamics. I do not mean, however, to give the impression that Browning has gathered around him a school of faithful disciples. Some have actually been quite critical of certain elements in his understanding of the moral dimension in pastoral care (Gerkin 1991, p.49; Graham 1996, ch.4). But they all agree that this dimension needs greater attention, both in theory and in practice.

Perhaps the most radical re-interpretation of pastoral care is that which seeks to incorporate socio-political analysis (Pattison 1994; Poling 1988, 1996). The logic is that as those who are involved in a pastoral ministry have a concern to relieve suffering, and as oppression and injustice are major causes of human suffering, it is necessary to be discerning pathways to liberation. While I believe that there is certainly a place for socio-political analysis within pastoral theology, it is important that the pastoral dimension is clearly identified and defined. Otherwise, pastoral theologians end up simply replicating, probably with less skill, the kind of work social ethicists are already doing. Socio-political inquiry will play a relatively small, but nonetheless significant, role in our investigations. Where I have embarked on such an inquiry, I hope I have been clear enough in my attempts to detail the pastoral implications.

The eminent American pastoral theologian Charles Gerkin has been another leader in the movement to 'widen the horizons' of pastoral theology. He has, for example, argued that the emotional climate or atmosphere of a town is a pastoral issue (Gerkin 1986). Christian leaders need, therefore, to be reflecting on how they might contribute to lifting the mood of their community. More recently, Gerkin has analysed moral and spiritual capacity in terms of three metaphors: 'presence', 'community' and 'vocation' (Gerkin 1991). His aim is to develop a moral interpretation of life which establishes 'normative boundaries for living' (Gerkin 1991, p.11). Presence refers to how we engage with others. Christians need to be shaping their way of being in relationship in order to reflect the love and grace of Christ. Interestingly, Gerkin also addresses the question of the way a whole congregation is present to its community. The second metaphor is an extension of the first. Gerkin observes that one of the most urgent needs in the modern world is for community. Finally, under the rubric of 'vocation' he addresses the issue of how believers respond to God's call to serve others through their gifts and abilities.

On the British scene, Alastair Campbell has produced an interesting and challenging theological interpretation of human service (Campbell 1984). He describes quite beautifully the mutuality in professional caring relationships through the use of the words 'gift', 'gratitude' and 'grace'. Both the human service provider and the client give gifts in the experience they share in. The relationship reaches its full potential when both are able to receive that which is offered with gratitude and grace. At that point, both have expressed a 'moderated love'. This is a real love, but it is a love that operates within the boundaries established in the professional environment.

More recently, the English practical theologian Elaine Graham has argued that we must take seriously the postmodern world we live in and the enormous challenges it poses to the emotional and spiritual well-being of individuals. 'The subject of care,' she observes, 'is shifting from that of a selfactualized individual for whom care functions primarily at times of crisis towards one of a person in need of nurture and support as she or he negotiates a complexity of moral and theological challenges in a rapidly-changing economic and social context' (Graham 1996, p.51). The postmodern world does indeed move at a fast pace, and more and more pastoral work will take the form of assisting people in negotiating the moral and spiritual challenges thrown at them.

In line with the general approach to pastoral theology that I have just described, I am seeking to identify certain key elements in an interpretation of relationships in human service provision and in organisational life which may be assigned a normative status. It is my intention to describe in spiritual and ethical terms some of the factors which contribute to the flourishing of those who inhabit this world. Put differently, I am interested in using a religio-ethical framework to discern the conditions in human service acts and in the organisational life supporting those acts which enhance the well-being of the various actors. In developing this framework, I am seeking to address two audiences. First, I am aiming to make a contribution to the ongoing task of broadening the horizons of pastoral theology. That is, I hope that what I have to say will inform the thought and action of professional theologians, pastors and lay leaders. It is also my hope, however, that my reflections will be of use to people who grapple daily with the task of spiritualising life in their professional worlds. Though there are some technical ethical and theological discussions, I hope that readers without expertise in these areas will nevertheless be able to find new perspectives on their attempts to promote the good in their professional environments.

In the first part of the book, our attention is directed to certain human service professions, namely nursing, midwifery, education and psychotherapy. The central religio-ethical concept that we will be working with is *self-communication*. It is a term which expresses a particular form of neighbour love: one which involves a donation of one's personal gifts and resources in order to meet a need in the other. The meeting of that need may require a personal involvement through compassion, empathy, warmth, support and affirmation. I will be suggesting that, for those engaged in personal service, charm is also an important element in self-communication. In my understanding, while charm is associated with an engaging and attractive presence, it is also something deeper. Following the French philosopher Gabriel Marcel, I construe it as a personal presence which refreshes the spirit of the other, which helps her to know herself more fully. Taking an 'aretaic' line on ethics (the Greek word *arete* indicates inner excellence and refers to the cultivation of virtue), the central argument in the first half of the book is that self-communication is a virtue in the human service professions. When those engaged in human service have a high capacity for self-communication, they contribute to the well-being of those in their care in a way that complements and completes their technical input.

In the second part, we will shift our focus from the spirituality of human service acts to the moral quality of the organisational life that is the context for those acts. The aim is to see how the insights of organisational theorists concerning intelligent workplace relations apply in the particular case of human service provision.

The key motifs in the discussion will be *belonging* and *trust*. Those in management tend to interpret a sense of belonging and the presence of trust in terms of efficiency. They view them as forms of 'social capital' which contribute to organisational effectiveness. Our concern, however, is primarily a pastoral one. When the various actors in the workplace feel at home in their environments and operate (most of the time at least) in relationships characterised by trust, they will tend to flourish. It is important, then, to identify those factors which produce belonging and trust. As I have just indicated, organisational theory is one significant resource in this search. Given the fact that belonging and trust are central facts in the *covenant life* described in the Hebrew and Christian scriptures, a second source suggests itself. It is through the dialogue between these two sources that our understanding of the conditions which promote the well-being of the actors in organisational life will be generated.

In sum, the three central terms in this book – self-communication, belonging and trust – have a very important place both in religio-ethical discussions and in cultural interpretations of human service and of organisational life. Through a process of cross-fertilisation, I aim to construct a model of the attitudes and behaviours which contribute to psychological and spiritual well-being in the human service world.

PART I

Self-Communication in the Human Service Professions

Introduction to Part I

In this first part, the major aim is to show that self-communication is a virtue in the human service professions. In choosing four particular professions for attention – nursing, midwifery, education and psychotherapy – I am aware that my selections may seem arbitrary. I could have, for example, included medicine, occupational therapy and social work. My aim, however, is not to be comprehensive, but rather to illustrate through reference to these four professions the value of self-communication in human service.

In the Introduction, I referred to the concept of self-communication in very general terms. It is now necessary to describe it more precisely. Self-communication involves two actions. First, there is an attempt to imaginatively grasp the thoughts, feelings, values, hopes and aspirations of the other. That is, one tries to discern the nature of the claim the other is making. Second, one responds to that claim through the giving of one's personal gifts and resources. In order to flesh out this description, I will make use of the teachings of the so-called 'dialogical' philosophers Martin Buber and Gabriel Marcel. These existentialist thinkers (although Marcel, at least, did not like being referred to as an existentialist) reflected on the nature of the dialogue between two individuals and developed certain crucial categories to describe it. An imaginative entry into the inner world of the other Buber calls 'inclusion'; answering the claims of the other he calls 'responsibility'. Marcel's term for putting oneself at the disposal of the other is *disponibilité*. It may be translated as 'availability' or 'disposability'. Availability involves both a reception of the person of the other, and a belonging to her in which one is prepared to substitute her freedom for one's own. In the first chapter, we will discuss these dialogical concepts in some depth.

Chapters 2 and 3 are devoted to the attempt to show that self-communication is a virtue in human service. The way that I will go about this is to set the idea of a virtue in the context of Alasdair MacIntyre's notion of a 'practice'. A practice is (roughly) a co-operative form of activity in which participants activate their excellences to achieve together the goods inherent in that particular practice. For MacIntyre, the virtues may be thought of (at least in a partial way) as those dispositions which sustain a practice and facilitate the attainment of the internal goods associated with it. In order to show that it is appropriate to refer to self-communication as a virtue in the human service practices, it is necessary to discuss how particular expressions of self-giving function as excellences which move persons towards certain key ends established for those practices. My argument will be that it is in and through presence, compassion, empathy and affirmation that some of the principal goods associated with human service are attained.

There is another form of self-communication which is hardly ever, if at all, associated with human service, and that is charm. We will discuss its role in Chapter 4. Following Marcel, I will construe charm as a personal presence which refreshes the soul of the other and reveals her self more deeply to herself. While I would agree that charm should not be rated as highly in importance as the other expressions of self-giving – empathy, compassion and affirmation – I suggest that neither should its value be under-estimated. Charm is a significant factor in promoting the well-being of others. Under its influence, persons are able to engage with life with renewed vigour, joy and hope.

I hope that the broad outlines of the discussion in the first half of the book are now in view. We will begin that discussion by attempting to gain a comprehensive understanding of self-communication.

CHAPTER 1

Self-Communication

The agapic approach to life is characterised by a willingness to give of one's self in meeting the needs of others. Those needs, of course, vary. They may be of a material, physical, emotional, intellectual or spiritual nature. We will not concern ourselves here with the first category. But in considering the human service professions I have chosen to work with, namely nursing, midwifery, education and psychotherapy, we are concerned with all the other dimensions of human need. Those for whom their vocation is human service, I will be arguing in subsequent chapters, are called to communication of the self in meeting the existential needs of others. Self-communication in a relationship, I suggest, refers to the desire and the capacity to, first, imaginatively enter the inner domain of the thoughts, feelings, values, hopes and aspirations of the other and so to interpret the nature of her claim, and, then, to make available the best of one's personal gifts and resources in responding to that claim.

In the dialogical thought of Martin Buber and Gabriel Marcel we find rich and insightful interpretations of self-communication. To describe the process of imaginatively grasping the attitudes, convictions, needs and aspirations of the other, Buber coined the term 'inclusion'. In including one's-self (the term Marcel employs to communicate the notion of the self that one is – the self which one makes available to others) in the inner world of another, one becomes aware of the claim she is making. The action of offering oneself in responding to that claim he called 'responsibility'. The third key notion associated with self-communication, at least as I have defined it, is 'availability'. It is a translation of Gabriel Marcel's term *disponibilité*. In this chapter, I will attempt to develop a comprehensive understanding of self-communication through a discussion of *inclusion, responsibility* and *availability*.

Inclusion

In his early writings, Buber (1947) refers to inclusion as 'experiencing the other side'. In order to describe what he means, he uses somatic analogies. Think, for example, of a person striking another. For a moment, he may be able to imagine what it feels like to receive that blow. In that passing moment, he experiences the situation from the other side. Or, alternatively, think of a woman caressing a man. She may be able to feel the contact from two sides: with the palm of her hand and also with the man's skin. Such inclusiveness 'is the complete realization of the submissive person, the desired person, the "partner", not by the fancy but by the actuality of the being' (Buber 1947, p.97). Thus, it is an entering into the experience of the other in a deep way – with one's body, mind and soul fully engaged.

Inclusion, according to Buber, has both 'abstract' and 'concrete' forms. The former he illustrates with reference to two persons engaged in a disputation (Buber 1947, p.99). They have a very different vision of life, of the world. At first, they are preoccupied with their own arguments. But then, in an instant, each one becomes aware of the other's 'full legitimacy' as a person. There is an immediate grasp of the spiritual dimension which grounds the other in 'the Present Being'. This represents, then, contact with the source of both his particularity and his validation as a person. Buber uses the word 'abstract' to describe this experience because while there is a recognition of the other as a spiritual being, there is no swinging into his concrete experience of life (very little may be known of this).

When Buber (1947, p.100) turns his attention to the educative process, however, he suggests that a *concrete* form of inclusion is required. The educator, says Buber, must be over there, standing with the student she is communicating with, as well as standing in her place on the rostrum. It is not enough to simply grasp the spiritual dimension in the student, as important as this is; the teacher must also be able to concretely feel what it is like to be taught. The inclusion, however (as, one might add, in the counselling context), is not mutual: '[The teacher] stands at both ends of the common situation, the pupil only at one end. In the moment when the pupil is able to throw herself across and experience from over there, the educative relation would be burst asunder, or change into friendship' (Buber 1947, p.100).

This last observation is quite important for our discussion of the human service professions. It is necessary for a person engaged in personal service to imaginatively place herself in the situation of the client. She needs to be able to sense what it is like to be at the other end of her nursing care, her teaching, or her therapeutic interventions, as the case may be. In this way, she assesses whether she is really meeting the needs of the client. But it is neither necessary nor appropriate for the client to think and feel herself into the experience of the service provider. There may be a certain kind of mutuality in the relationship in that the patient or student may communicate something of herself that is enriching to the professional working with her. This mutuality, however, does not extend to the act of inclusion. Two-way inclusion belongs only to friendship.

To those of us familiar with counselling theory, the notion of 'inclusion' sounds very much like empathy. But, for Buber, empathy in the strictest sense involves a loss of contact with one's own thoughts and feelings which has no part in inclusion:

> [Empathy] means to 'transpose' oneself over there and in there. Thus it means the exclusion of one's own concreteness, the extinguishing of the actual situation of life, the absorption in pure aestheticism of the reality in which one participates. Inclusion is the opposite of this. It is the extension of one's own concreteness, the fulfilment of the actual situation of life, the complete presence of the reality in which one participates. (Buber 1947, p.97)

The reason Buber emphasises the importance of maintaining one's 'concreteness' is that dialogue between an 'I' and a 'thou' requires both persons to be fully present. In her uniqueness and particularity as a person, the I enters into the 'otherness' of the thou, into his particular expression of personhood, and vice versa. If either partner loses contact with their concreteness, there is no possibility of a genuine meeting. There needs to be, then, a 'mutual recognition' which establishes dialogue.

> To recognize means for us creatures the fulfilment by each of us, in truth and responsibility, of his own relation to the Present Being, through our receiving all that is manifested of it and incorporating it into our own being, with all our force, faithfully, and open to the world and the spirit. (Buber 1947, p.99)

To our meeting we bring our own particular way of engaging with life, of participating in Being. In order to enter into a genuine dialogue, we need to recognise each other's unique way of being in the world.

I agree that one must maintain contact with, and give full expression to, one's personhood in relating to the other. I accept, also, that in a deep empathic engagement one may temporarily lose contact with one's concrete personal reality. Consider, for example, Carl Rogers' (1980) view that to enter the private world of the other

> means that for the time being, you lay aside your own views and values... In some sense it means that you lay aside yourself; this can only be done by persons who are secure enough in themselves that they know they will not get lost in what may turn out to be the strange and bizarre world of the other, and that they can comfortably return to their own world when they wish. (p.143)

It is my view, however, that to refer to empathy and inclusion as 'opposites' is to make too much of the difference between the two. After all, as Rogers points out, one can return at will to one's own reality in order to communicate it to the other.

In his later writings, Buber (1957) used terms such as 'personal making present' and 'imagining the real' to describe this process in which one imaginatively enters the inner domain of the other. In order to enter into a relation with a person it is necessary to become aware of the other as 'a whole, as a unity, and as unique' (p.109). When I am aware of him in this way he becomes present to me. I have managed to grasp something of 'the dynamic center which stamps his every utterance, action, and attitude with the recognizable sign of uniqueness' (p.109). Reaching into the inner domain of another in this way involves an act of the imagination. 'Imagining the real' is 'not a looking at the other, but a bold swinging, demanding the most intensive stirring of the one's being, into the life of the other' (p.110).

Responsibility

This awareness of the other through which he becomes present in his wholeness and uniqueness Buber (1947, pp.8–10) contrasts with two other perceptual modes, namely 'observing' and 'looking on'. The observer operates with a quasi-scientific mindset. She is interested in a careful, analytical study of the other. Her aim is to compile a comprehensive list of traits. For the purposes of observation, the other person is nothing but a bundle of characteristics.

The onlooker is not at all interested in traits. Focusing on traits, he thinks, leads one away from one's real purpose. Looking on – the artistic perspective – involves trusting one's intuitive powers. That which is really significant about the other will show itself if only one is attentive and receptive.

Neither in observing or in looking on, however, do we find the possibility of being addressed directly by the other. The observer perceives a bundle of traits, the onlooker an existence, but the one who is *aware* perceives a call to action, feels the weight of destiny falling on him:

> [I]n a receptive hour of my personal life a man meets me about whom there is something, which I cannot grasp in any objective way at all, that 'says something' to me. That does not mean, says to me what manner of man this is, what is going on in him, and the like. But it means, says something to me, addresses something *to me*, speaks something that enters my own life. (Buber 1947, p.9)

In becoming aware that I have been addressed, I have a moral obligation to respond. 'Responsibility presupposes one who addresses me primarily, that is, from a realm independent of myself, and to whom I am answerable. He addresses me about something that he has entrusted to me and that I am bound to take care of loyally' (Buber 1947, p.45).

In order to answer the claims the other makes, one must be inclined to generously make available one's personal resources. The person who is self-absorbed, who tends to cling to herself, cannot possibly respond. To describe a willingness to make the self available, Gabriel Marcel uses the word *disponibilité*. It has a financial connotation and is linked to the notion of disposable assets. The available person is the one who is prepared to put all of her assets at the disposal of the other.

Availability

Marcel (1964a) also interprets *disponibilité* in terms of receptivity. He develops the link between the two terms in an essay in *Creative Fidelity* entitled 'Phenomenological Notes on Being in a Situation'. To exist with others, he observes, is to be exposed to influences. It is not possible to be human without to some extent being permeable to those influences. Permeability, in its broadest sense, is associated with a certain lack of cohesion or density. Thus, the fact of being exposed to external influences is linked with a kind of *incohesion*. I am 'porous', open to a reality which seeks to communicate with me. Marcel (1964a) puts it this way:

> I must somehow make room for the other in myself; if I am completely absorbed in myself, concentrated on my sensations, feelings, anxieties, it will obviously be impossible for me to receive, to incorporate in myself, the message of the other. What I called incohesion a moment ago here assumes the form of disposability. (p.88)

Disposability, then, is closely associated with receptivity. Receptivity involves a readiness to make available one's personal centre, one's ownmost domain. We receive others in a room, in a house, or in a garden, but not on unknown ground or in the woods. Receptivity means that I invite the other *chez soi* (Marcel 1950, p.118). That is, I invite him to 'be at home' with me. A home receives the imprint of one's personality; something of myself is infused into the way my home space is constructed. Contrast this with 'the nameless sadness' associated with a hotel room; this is no one's home. To share one's home space is disposability or availability because '[t]o provide hospitality is truly to communicate something of oneself to the other' (Marcel 1950, p.91).

The meaning of hospitality can also be broadened to include receiving into oneself the appeal of another for understanding and compassion. When I open myself to the call of the other to be with her in her pain and confusion, I am able to spontaneously feel with her. The intonation of my words, my facial expressions and perhaps my tears all say to her that I am with her in her suffering. Contrasted to this responsiveness, however, there is an indisposability which Marcel refers to as an 'inner inertia' or 'spiritual asthenia' (Marcel 1964b, p.50). The distress of the other is experienced as something alien; I simply cannot receive it into my ownmost sphere. To illustrate this fundamental lack of responsiveness, Marcel (1964b, pp.50–51) contrasts the mundane scenario of a person asking for information which is not at one's disposal with the case of a person appealing to one's sympathy. In the first case, I must respond to a concrete question such as, 'What is the population of Rome?' I go through my 'file' of information and find that there is nothing available in relation to this question. Marcel (1964b) then moves to the appeal for understanding:

> Here again I must furnish a response but it will be of a completely different kind; it could turn out that this response which involves my

feeling is not within my power to draw out of myself. I do not succeed in summoning forth the sympathy which is entreated. I would have wished it to be otherwise and it is painful to deceive my questioner, but what can I do? I can only utter certain formulas I have in mind which are part of my repertory and seem to suit the present circumstances; perhaps I can find it possible to give them a sympathetic intonation, but in any case I am only reading something out of a catalogue; this reaction is relevant only to having as in the case of the file above; it has nothing in common with that positive human sympathy to which the other person appeals and which I really do not feel. The suffering of the other person is alien to me and I do not succeed in making it my own. (pp.50–51)

The only way to break out of this 'self-obsession', according to Marcel (1964b), is by 'submerging oneself suddenly in the life of another person and being forced to see things through his eyes' (p.51). One cannot break out of this 'inner inertia' on one's own; it is through the presence of another person that this 'miracle' is accomplished. The miracle does not, of course, happen automatically; one must be open, responsive, to the appeal of the other.

We are, however, still left with the questions: 'Why am I non-responsive to the suffering of the other?' 'Why do I feel opaque, non-permeable?' Marcel believes that non-availability is associated with the tendency to see one's existence in terms of possession. I will treat myself as indisposable 'just so far as I construe my life or being as a having which is somehow quantifiable, hence as something capable of being wasted, exhausted or dissipated' (Marcel 1964b, p.54). In this attitude, I become like a person who knows that his small sum of money must last a very long time. I become afflicted with an anxiety and a concern which discourages self-giving. These negative affects are 'reabsorbed into a state of inner inertia' (Marcel 1964b, p.54).

But if we feel we really belong to another person, we do not count the cost of, or keep a score on, our self-communication. Marcel broadened his analysis of availability to include the idea of belonging. We seem to be on dangerous ground in speaking about belonging to another person. It seems as if I must disenfranchise myself in giving myself away. Do I not in this act give up my personal autonomy? Marcel (1964b) is acutely aware of the pitfalls associated with conceiving of disposability in terms of belonging. He begins his analysis with the case of servanthood. If I assert, he says, of a servant 'he belongs to me', I treat him as a thing acquired, as something to be disposed of as I wish. Everything changes, though, if I declare to another person 'I belong to you'. 'Jack, I belong to you' means 'I am opening an unlimited credit account in your name, you can do what you want with me, I give myself to you' (Marcel 1964b, p.40). As the moral theologian Robert Gibbs observes, the use of a name, 'Jack', is important here (Gibbs 1989). I am speaking to a unique person, to a *thou*. The claims associated with belonging can only be communicated in the first person.

The fact that I give myself to you does not mean that I am your slave. I establish my freedom in the very act of freely giving myself to you. '[T]he best use I can make of my freedom is to place it in your hands; it is as though I freely substituted your freedom for my own; or paradoxically, it is by that very substitution that I realize my freedom' (Marcel 1964b, p.40). (Here we are reminded of Jesus' teaching on gain through loss. See, for example, Mk 8:35; Mk 9:35; Jn 12:24.)

Though Marcel can assert that to give oneself freely to the other is to be free indeed, he feels the need to establish how it is possible that one can substitute the freedom of another for one's own without a disenfranchisement. In order to give one's-self freely, one must have some authority over the self that is given. That is to say, if I am to dispose of myself I must belong to myself. In an attempt to understand what it means to speak of a belonging to self, Marcel (1964b, pp.42–46) develops the highly original notion of the self as constituted by an older and a younger brother. He begins with the (inadequate) idea that I treat myself as an object belonging to the subject that I at the same time am. The difficulty here is that 'I' is the very negation of objectivity. In adopting the formulation 'object belonging to the subject I at the same time am', one is really saying that the 'I' can be treated as a 'him', which is of course meaningless in this context. It is evident, then, that the 'I belong to myself' must be *personalised*. In this way, I can say that 'I have custody over myself or I am a trustee of myself' (Marcel 1964b, p.42). Belonging to myself means that I am responsible for myself, and this seems to suggest that I am two persons. It is as if I am at once the older and the younger brother of myself. Marcel has in mind two orphaned brothers, with the older one being responsible for the younger one. When one begins to think this way, it is possible to construct a relational triad in which mutual availability and personal autonomy can co-exist. The components in this triad are these: 'I belong to you'; 'you belong to me'; 'I belong to myself' (Marcel 1964b, p.42).

In a more conventional fashion, the theologian Alistair McFadyen arrives at the same conclusion in his Christian theory of personhood and relationships (McFadyen 1990). Crucial to the formation of personhood is what McFadyen calls 'being centred'. The centring of one's experience in the self is what constitutes autonomy. Being centred is defined as the 'achievement of organising one's life from an organisational locus within oneself; the ability to refer the features of the world to oneself and one's own location, so that the possibilities for action may be focussed on as they relate to oneself and so be self-ascribed' (McFadyen 1990, p.312). I refer my experience of the world to my personal centre and thereby ensure that my actions are self-ascribed. This is another way of stating Marcel's idea that 'I belong to myself'. The normative pattern for dialogue, in McFadyen's (1990) schema, is built on the understanding that 'we are properly centred as persons only by being directed towards the true reality of other personal centres: we become truly ourselves when we are truly for others' (p.151). In Marcel's language, I avoid the self-constricting egoism potentially associated with the 'I belong to myself' when I simultaneously assert that 'I belong to you' and 'you belong to me'.

McFadyen points to the fact that in a Christian understanding mutual giving in a relationship is grounded in the presence and power of Christ. It is the grace of his sustaining love, appropriated through faith, which allows us to risk ourselves with others:

> The otherness of other people, including their brokenness, does not pose a threat of disintegration for those who live in the knowledge that they are upheld as integral beings in the presence of Christ, the indwelling of the Holy Spirit and in the love and acceptance of God and/or others: who are, in other words, empowered by the Spirit, conformed to Christ and called into responsibility before God and others. (McFadyen 1990, p.157)

In Marcel's (1964a) terminology, belonging to others is grounded in a belonging to Christ (pp.99–101). He acknowledges that there may be an initial revolt against Christ's claim that I belong to him. It seems as if I am losing myself in accepting his lordship. On the contrary, says Marcel, in Christ I am truly free. The person of faith knows that Christ is not really someone else but 'more internal to me than myself' (Marcel 1964a, p.100). His right is exercised not in terms of power but of love. If I can but overcome my unproductive resistance to what seems a tyrannical claim, I am set free from the strangulating grip of egoism.

> [W]ho am I to pretend that I do not belong to You? The point really is that if I belong to You, this doesn't mean: I am Your possession; this mysterious relation does not exist on the level of having as would be the case if You were an infinite power. Not only are You freedom, but You also will me, You arouse me too as freedom, You invite me to create myself, You are this very invitation. And if I reject it, i.e. Thou, if I persist in maintaining that I belong only to myself, it is as though I walled myself up; as though I strove to strangle with my own hands that reality in whose name I believed I was resisting You. (Marcel 1964a, p.100)

I belong to myself; I belong to Christ; I belong to you; you belong to me. With these statements, Marcel creatively constructs an understanding of availability which holds together personal autonomy and freedom on the one hand, and genuine giving of the self to others and to Christ on the other. Christ is the ground of the free act in which I substitute your freedom for mine, just as you substitute mine for yours.

Self-communication, Marcel and universal love

I said at the beginning of this chapter that the agapic life requires a commitment to employ one's gifts and resources in meeting the needs of the other. In this way, I was suggesting that self-communication is an expression of *agape*. That the two notions are very closely linked was made abundantly clear in the last section when we incorporated the concept of availability. When Marcel makes the claim that availability involves belonging to the other, he seems to be on dangerous ground. In his statement 'I am opening an unlimited credit account in your name, you can do what you want with me, I give myself to you', he appears to be advocating a radical form of agapic love in which the well-being of the self is dismissed as having little or no importance. By contrast, a number of moral and pastoral theologians have posited an understanding of love, variously called impartiality, equal-regard or universal love, which assigns equal importance to other-regard and to self-regard (Browning 1987, 1992; Janssens 1977; Outka 1972, 1992). That is, the protection and advancement of the well-being of the self and of the other are given the same priority. As Browning (1987) observes, the tendency within Christianity to promote self-denying altruism has been challenged by both those with a therapeutic awareness and those with a justice orientation. There are those, first, who have strenuously insisted that good mental health requires an appropriate self-love. Each person has certain physical, emotional and intellectual needs which she must attend to if she is to flourish. And, second, there are those thinkers who have argued that the ideal of self-denial has been used as a tool by those in positions of power and privilege to control those in subordinate groups. In this way, women, blacks and others have been hoodwinked into giving up their claims on a fulfilling and satisfying life in order that the elites may maintain their position.

With these strong challenges before us, it is easy to see why many moral thinkers want to assign an equal rank to self- and other-regard. According to the principle of impartiality or equal-regard, one should love the other neither less nor more than oneself. Outka (1992) prefers the concept of what he calls 'universal love' because, though it is closely associated with impartiality, it also moves beyond it to incorporate the Christian commitment to being for the other. I want to discuss briefly Outka's analysis because I contend that it has close links with Marcel's interpretation of availability. While it may seem that at certain points Marcel has scant regard for self-love, a comprehensive survey of his writings indicates that he in fact sought to balance regard for the other with regard for the self.

Outka (1992) lists four challenges to the principle of impartiality. It is the first two that are particularly relevant to our discussion. First, impartiality cannot find a place for the radically other-regarding elements in *agape*. Second, it does not take seriously the fact that we are more likely to be tempted by selfishness than by altruism. Outka is prepared to align himself with impartiality to the extent that altruism is not given an endorsement if it is of the radical kind which is dismissive of self-love. However, in taking these two objections seriously, he suggests that it is necessary to go beyond impartiality and incorporate 'a practical swerve' away from self and towards the other. Given the fact that we have great difficulty in being even-handed when it comes to balancing our own needs against those of the other, we need to build in a bias towards her well-being.

Outka's proposal is attractive because it acknowledges that the needs of the self do matter, while offering a way to counteract the deep-seated temptation to selfishness which mitigates other-regard. I suggest that Marcel's understanding of availability is actually quite close to Outka's idea of universal love. As I have said, Marcel, in his statement that belonging to the other one means that one gives him the right to do what he wants, seems to be advocating a submission to exploitation. The statement, however, must be taken in the context of a mutual commitment to belonging. The unreserved offering of self – 'I belong to you; do with me as you will' – assumes an identical intention from the other. Further, Marcel does include a discussion on the role of self-love within his reflections on availability as belonging. His treatment ends with a statement which, I believe, is clearly in support of the principle of universal love. To begin with, he defines self-love as a 'charity towards oneself' (Marcel 1964b, p.46). The self is to be thought of as 'a seed which must be cultivated, as a ground which must be readied for the spiritual or even the divine in this world' (Marcel 1964b, p.46). This nurture of the self requires patience. Harshness towards the self stunts growth. But in being patient one is also 'lucid' in relation to the self. That is, self-love does not come with a licence to overlook one's moral failings and defects. Self-love, properly understood, incorporates both 'distance from and nearness to the self' (Marcel 1964b, p.46). In maintaining distance from ourselves we are able to see clearly the areas we need to work on to strengthen our capacity for love of neighbour. Nearness to ourselves means that we have a 'contact with ourselves that we should always have with our fellow-men' (Marcel 1964b, p.47). That is, we should show the same charity to ourselves as we do to our neighbours.

'Nearness to self' expresses the importance of an appropriate self-love. Marcel does not demand that we treat the self as if it is of little or no importance. On the other hand, 'distance from self' involves the recognition that we are often blind to our selfishness and need to attempt to reflect 'lucidly' on our commitment to others. The 'distance' pole in Marcel's analysis is, I suggest, his way of advocating a 'practical swerve' away from self in the direction of the other. Thus, he argues for a universal love.

Using the insights generated by Buber and Marcel, we have developed a rich understanding of what it means to include oneself in the inner domain of the other, and to respond to her claims through communicating something of one's self. In the rest of this first half of the book, the aim will be to show that self-communication is a virtue in the human service professions. A first step is to develop an understanding of aretaic ethics in general and of Alasdair MacIntyre's notion of a practice in particular.

CHAPTER 2

Virtue and Practices

It is evident that self-communication in relationships has an ethical dimension. A person's way of being with others can be evaluated in terms of right, wrong, obligation and the good. McClendon (1986, p.107) makes the interesting suggestion that a capacity for genuine presence in relationships is a virtue. He is content, however, to simply offer the insight in passing. It is a view which warrants exploration and development. The way in which I want to develop it is to construe self-giving in a people-oriented calling as a virtue. In order to do this, I will make use of Alasdair MacIntyre's work on virtues and practices. The task in this chapter is to describe that work.

In the next chapter, the aim will be to show how self-communication in one's profession, virtue and MacIntyre's (1985) notion of a practice all fit together. We will see below precisely how MacIntyre defines a practice. Here the concept may be introduced by saying that a practice is (roughly) a co-operative form of activity in which participants activate their 'excellences' to achieve together the goods inherent in that particular activity. For MacIntyre, the virtues may be thought of (at least in a partial way) as those dispositions which sustain a practice and facilitate the attainment of the internal 'goods' (i.e. 'inherent moral values') associated with it. In order to show that it is appropriate to refer to self-communication as a virtue (at least in MacIntyre's sense), it is necessary to discuss how particular expressions of authentic being-with function as excellences which move persons towards the ends established for a particular practice. It is natural to look to places such as the hospital, the school and the psychotherapist's office in search of activities where self-communication might be considered a virtue. (The church is obviously another place to look. For a treatment of pastoral availability, see Pembroke 2002.) This we will do in the following chapter.

To return to the assignment for this chapter, a necessary starting point is setting MacIntyre's work on virtue and the virtues in some sort of context. Up until relatively recently in the field of ethics, there have been two major emphases. On the one hand, there have been those who have been committed to an approach focused on the rules and principles describing moral duty. Since the Greek word *deon* means 'duty', this is known as the 'deontological' approach. On the other hand, there are those moral philosophers who stress the need to assess the outcome or any moral decision in terms of the ratio of good over evil that is likely to result from it. That is, they are interested in the probable consequences attaching to moral decision making. The term used to describe this school of thought is 'teleological' (*telos* means 'aim' or 'end'). Due, in part, to widespread dissatisfaction with the deontological and teleological perspectives, there has been a resurgence of interest in the way the categories of virtue and character may be profitably employed in moral thinking. In order to establish the place of virtue or aretaic ethics in contemporary moral philosophy, it will be necessary to set it beside its competitors. (The term 'aretaic' is applied to virtue ethics because *arete* refers to the excellence that is associated with a strong moral character.)

Given that MacIntyre, like virtually all other virtue ethicists, makes significant use of Aristotle and Aquinas, it is important that we gain some understanding of their thought. Aquinas used many of the concepts developed by his teacher, but he added a theological dimension. Further, he found an important place in his schema for a human capacity that Aristotle all but ignored, namely the will. In discussing the work of these great philosophers, we will be laying the foundations for an understanding of MacIntyre's work. Our first task, however, is to analyse the rival systems to virtue ethics.

The resurgence in virtue ethics

Prior to the Enlightenment period, moral philosophy was orientated to natural law and the idea of virtue. In the modern period, however, deontological and teleological theories have moved to centre stage. Due, in part, to dissatisfaction with these approaches, there has been something of a resurgence of interest in virtue and character as important categories for moral theory. Here the recovery of virtue ethics is set in the context of a general description of its competitors. There have been a large number of theories developed which are either rule- or goal-based. Each of the theories has a different emphasis, and the differences are sometimes quite subtle. It is not necessary here to follow every twist and turn in the different approaches. Rather, riding over the broad contours will set the resurgence of virtue ethics in some sort of context. Since classical utilitarianism emerged out of a dissatisfaction with natural law theory, it is with the latter that we begin.

Natural law theories, whether in the Stoic, Thomist (the approach of the most eminent of the medieval Christian philosopher-theologians, Thomas Aquinas) or some other version, are all grounded in the view that from a study of nature in general and of human nature in particular it is possible to generate precepts applicable to all persons at all times. 'There is in fact a true law – namely right reason – which is in accordance with nature,' wrote Cicero, 'applies to all men, and is unchangeable and eternal. By its commands this law summons men to the performance of their duties; by its prohibitions it restrains them from doing wrong' (*De Republica*, II, 22; cited in Kainz 1988, p.70).

As Kainz (1988) points out, a commitment to an eternal and unchanging law of nature is built on a view of nature as stable. It is evident that if nature is changing rapidly and in an unpredictable fashion, the theory is thrown into confusion. Further, natural law theory can only survive if the theories of nature supporting it are also stable. As soon as the consensus in the theories breaks down, the whole project is undermined. In an attempt to work down to a solid bedrock for moral theory, thinkers such as Hobbes, Locke and Rousseau began to investigate the condition of humanity in its natural state; that is, before it was affected by the civilisation process. However, what emerged was not a unified theory of the state of nature, but rather a number of very different accounts of the human values and behaviours which are presumed to be natural to the human person. There were those thinkers who wanted to maintain an empirical stance, but who wanted to find a way around the uncertainties and pitfalls associated with the quest for the human's original natural state. Jeremy Bentham, for example, thought that the principle of social utility would furnish the requisite objectivity and certainty:

> Nature has placed mankind under the governance of two sovereign masters, *pain* and *pleasure*. The *principle of utility* recognizes this

subjection... An action may be said to be conformable to the principle of utility...when the tendency it has to augment the happiness of the community is greater than any it has to diminish it. (Bentham 1970, ch. II, p.xiv; cited in Kainz 1988, p.78)

The basic criterion of what is morally right, wrong or obligatory in utilitarian theories is the *consequences* which flow from particular rules or acts. That is, they have a teleological frame of reference. The ultimate end posited is the greatest general good. A rule or action is right if, and only if, it can be assessed as likely to produce at least as great a balance of good over evil for the community as a whole as any alternative (Frankena 1963). It is important to recognise that the good referred to here is non-moral good: food, shelter, health, etc.

Against this commitment to the principle of utility, deontologists argue that there are other considerations which take precedence over the goodness or badness of consequences. That is to say, there are certain universal principles which establish what is right or obligatory. It is therefore possible, they argue, for an action or rule to be morally right or obligatory even if it doesn't promote the greatest possible ratio of good over evil.

A standard objection to rule-based moral theory is that there are always exceptions to any rule. Consider a basic moral rule such as 'Always tell the truth'. It is possible to find oneself in a situation where one needs to make an exception to this rule in order to promote a good greater than absolute honesty. For example, Tom knows where Fred, a friend, is at this moment. Ed arrives at Tom's house and inquires about Fred's whereabouts. Tom, however, is aware that Ed intends to harm his friend. In order to protect him, Tom must lie. The principle 'Always tell the truth' is in conflict in this case with the principle 'Protect others from harm when it is in one's power to do so'.

It is possible to avoid the problem of conflict between moral principles if it can be shown that there is only one basic principle. In constructing his famous categorical imperative, Immanuel Kant aims at identifying just such a principle: 'There is...but one categorical imperative, namely this: *Act only on that maxim whereby thou canst at the same time will that it should become a universal law...*' (Kant 1949, p.38; emphasis in the original). Here Kant is saying two things. First, when one acts voluntarily one always acts in terms of a maxim or rule which can be formulated. And second, one's action can be evaluated as genuinely moral if, and only if, one would be prepared to universalise one's maxim.

Whether the orientation is to a categorical imperative or social utility, the aim is to ground morality in a rational principle. In the Aristotelian schema the focus is on selfhood; now it has been shifted to universalisability and objectivity. MacIntyre (1985, ch.5) has persuasively argued that this whole Enlightenment project of grounding morality in rationality suffers from a fatal and inherent flaw. The Enlightenment moral thinkers, he points out, worked with a framework of moral reflection handed down to them by Aristotle and those who followed him. That is, their work had an historical determinant; it was embedded in a particular tradition of moral philosophy. The Aristotelian teleological scheme established the backdrop against which they worked out their own systems. This scheme has three elements: human nature in its morally uncultivated state, practical reason, and human nature shaped in accordance with its *telos* or aim. Thus, human nature in its untutored state is moved by practical reason to human nature shaped according to the *telos* of *eudaimonia* (happiness or blessedness). The Enlightenment moral theorists, however, rejected any notion of a *telos* for human nature. It is at this point, observes MacIntyre, that the fatal error creeps in. Aristotle's scheme is only coherent when all three elements are in place. Take one element out and the system collapses.

Michael Slote, also a virtue ethicist, finds another source of incoherence in this project of rationality for morality (Slote 1992, p.45). His attention is on Kantian ethics and on what he construes as its self–other asymmetry. In this modern age, notes Slote, with its robust commitment to self-affirmation, a self–other asymmetry in a moral system constitutes a weakness. There is in the Kantian scheme a duty on the moral agent to act so as to benefit others, but there is no such obligation to produce a benefit for herself. Kant argues that a person does not have a duty or obligation to pursue her own happiness simply because she will inevitably and spontaneously do so. When this claim, argues Slote, is linked with the assumption that the strength of our obligation to benefit others varies with the closeness of their relationship to us, it falls into incoherence. On the one hand, Kant would have it that we have a particularly strong obligation to seek the good of those closest to us (friends and family), but on the other hand he has it that we have no such obligation to seek our own good.

There have been numerous objections raised to utilitarian theory. Perhaps the most common is that it simply asks too much of the moral agent. While it is natural for a person to act in such a way as to promote her own happiness, it seems overly demanding to ask her at the same time to choose that course of action which will maximise the good of the majority. It is also commonly pointed out that the principle of social utility needs a principle of justice to lend it coherence. The classical utilitarian theory provides no way of arbitrating between, on the one hand, distributing a fixed amount of non-moral good to a small number of people and, on the other, distributing the same amount more widely.

For these and other reasons, some moral theorists have become dissatisfied with the prevailing theories and have decided to look again at the possibilities offered by an ethics of virtue. It is not, of course, that they are unaware of the difficulties associated with virtue ethics. A Kantian, for example, would contend that an ethics constructed around character is preoccupied with betterment of the moral agent, assigning too little importance to obligation and duty. There is also the problem of circularity in Aristotle's system. One becomes virtuous through repeated acts of virtue; but one can only act virtuously if one has an already firmly established character. That is, how does one break into the circle in the first place? How does one build up enough virtue to get the process of character formation going? Finally, in developing a moral system on the foundation of the notion of virtue, one must contend with the difficulty in establishing some unitary concept which ties together all the various expressions of what a virtue is. There are almost as many definitions of a virtue as there are theorists. Consequently, there is nothing like agreement on what a table of virtues should look like.

Despite these problems and difficulties, virtue ethicists have decided that their approach is, on balance, likely to be more fruitful than a reconstruction of existing deontological and/or utilitarian theories. While adopting a very different starting point to their competitors, they grant, however, that categories from these competing systems are important. They recognise that decision and obligation must have a place in any moral system, but they argue that vision rather than decision (Hauerwas 1981), and being rather than doing (Meilaender 1984), should take centre stage.

The duties we may see, the decisions we may make, depend on the virtues that shape our vision of the world. In building this alternative moral system, sooner or later most virtue ethicists find themselves returning to the foundational theories of Aristotle and Aquinas. In turning now to these central accounts, it is recognised that the business of interpreting these thinkers is a complicated and intricate affair. All that is necessary for our purposes, however, is to lay out as accurately as possible the key elements in their theories of the virtues.

Aristotle's theory of the virtues

Aristotle viewed human beings, along with all other creatures, as having a specific nature. Now it is in the nature of human beings and all other creatures to move towards a specific *telos* or goal. The human, then, has by nature an orientation to a good end. This good, says Aristotle, is *eudaimonia*. As is often the case with Greek, or any foreign language for that matter, finding precise correlates in English is often a problem. However, *eudaimonia* can be taken to mean happiness, blessedness, prosperity. MacIntyre (1985, p.148) expresses it well: 'It is the state of being well and doing well in being well, of a man's being well-favored himself and in relation to the divine.' The virtues are those dispositions which enable a person to attain *eudaimonia*, the lack of which will frustrate her movement towards that *telos*. Put simply, because of the way we are made we have a goal that we instinctively aim for – happiness – and the virtues we establish help us to get there.

A fundamental concern for Aristotle in his *Nichomachean Ethics* (hereafter referred to as *NE*; the text I have used is the Revised Oxford Translation – see Aristotle 1984) is to establish which division in the soul – passions, faculties or states – a virtue fits into. That is, he wants to know what kind of human capacity an excellence really is. What Aristotle calls the passions we would think of as emotional forces (e.g. love and fear). Though the emotional drives are important in the moral life, it is evident that much more is involved in the cultivation of virtue. So this first candidate gets ruled out. Our mental faculties, for their part, allow us to know that we are feeling this or that passion. But such a knowledge cannot take us to the heart of what it is to be virtuous. Thus, there is only one candidate left, namely the states. To be a person of moral character is to live in a state of virtue. Aristotle was a practical thinker, and as such he construed the virtues as capacities which helped a person do his or her work well. But they must also be viewed on another level. Not only do the excellences help us do good work, the primary fact is that they develop within us a *state* of goodness. We are able to do good work because we are virtuous persons.

> [E]very excellence both brings into good condition the thing of which it is an excellence and makes the work of that thing be done well... Therefore...the excellence of man also will be the state which makes a man good and which makes him do his own work well. (*NE* 1106a 15, 21)

Influencing and shaping the actions which flow out of a virtuous state is *pleasure* or *pain*.

> We must take as a sign of states the pleasure or pain that supervenes on acts; for the man who abstains from bodily pleasures and delights in this very fact is temperate, while the man who is annoyed at it is self-indulgent, and he who stands his ground against things that are terrible and delights in this or at least is not pained is brave, while the man who is pained is a coward. (*NE* 1104b 4–10)

This is, of course, a controversial element in Aristotle's theory. A Kantian, for example, would deny that moral action is in any way related to feelings. Remember that his emphasis is on *deon*, duty. The morally good person has the good will sufficient to do his duty simply because it is his duty. Nonetheless, it is a crucial element in Aristotle's account of moral excellence. In asserting the 'pleasure principle', he is rejecting the idea that the feelings associated with good and right acts are of no consequence in the moral life. A good person is the one who 'rejoice[s] in noble actions', who 'enjoy[s] acting justly' (*NE* 1099a 16–19). It is not enough, however, to describe the excellences of character in terms of feeling and desire. Action and truth are, according to Aristotle, also controlled by thought and *choice*. In a given situation requiring moral action, the virtuous person must choose how he will act in order to attain the good. Aristotle's theory of choice is involved and intricate. It is beyond the scope of this treatment of his work to pursue it fully. Here it is necessary only to sketch the broad outlines of his theory.

Choice is obviously linked to voluntariness. Aristotle observes that choice 'seems to be voluntary, but not all that is voluntary to be an object of choice. Is it, then, what has been decided on by previous deliberation? For choice involves reason and thought' (*NE* 1112a 15–17). Choice is 'deliberative desire of things in our power; for when we have decided as a result of deliberation, we desire in accordance with our deliberation' (*NE* 1113a 10–13). The expression 'deliberative desire' has important connotations, combining as it does the factors of rationality and feeling. Aristotle is very aware of the interdependence of reason and desire. Reason alone cannot move a person to act; a person turns his mind in a certain direction because he wants to. Desire alone is insufficient to determine conduct; it must be formed by reason. While Aristotle makes it clear that reason and desire are indissolubly linked in the context of action, he fails to state precisely how they relate to each other. It has been suggested that he needs the concept of intention to complete this segment of his theory. The idea of intention, that which relates to the *will* and not just to desire, allows us '[t]o describe the action of an uncontrolled man who has further intentions in doing what he does, whose actions are deliberate, although his deliberations are in the interests of a desire which conflicts with what he regards as doing well...' (Hauerwas 1975, p.54). What this means is that desire and will can be in conflict. There is a significant difference between saying that I have the *desire* to go for a one kilometre jog this afternoon, on the one hand, and that I *will* go for one, on the other. The exercise of will is more powerful than the presence of desire. We would all be better people if we could follow through on all our good intentions! Below we will see that Thomas Aquinas was very aware of this fact, and introduced the important component of will into his theory of virtue.

The capacity for making a good choice, it must also be noted, is possible because a person has attained the virtue of *practical wisdom* (*phronesis*). A person of practical wisdom possesses both true reasoning and right desire (*NE* 1139a 23–25). Reason and desire are harnessed in deliberating well in order to establish those passions and actions which conduce to the good life. In relation to passions and actions there is, observes Aristotle, excess, defect and the intermediate or *mean* (*NE* 1106b 16–28). It is possible to feel fear and confidence, anger and pity, and in general pleasure and pain too strongly or too weakly. Moral excellence, however, involves feeling the passions 'at the right times, with reference to the right objects, towards the right people, with the right aim, and in the right way' (NE 1106b 21–22). This is the intermediate. The situation is similar in relation to action. Judgement is required in matters pertaining to moral excellence to establish the mean. Thus the person possessing moral excellence and the capacity for right deliberation will establish courage as the mean between fear and rashness, liberality as the mean between prodigality and meanness, proper pride as sitting midway between empty vanity and undue humility, to name just a few of the possibilities.

The person of virtue uses reason to order and tame the passions and appetites. Reason can never be the slave of passion. The moral life is fundamentally about excellent deliberation ordering the passions and so moving the moral agent towards attainment of the good. Indeed, moral excellence and practical wisdom are indissolubly linked. Moral excellence establishes the right end for the human, and practical wisdom indicates the means for achieving that end (NE 1145a 4–6). Choice will not be right without both practical wisdom and moral excellence. It is not possible, therefore, for a person who is morally deficient to exercise practical wisdom. This Aristotle makes clear in an important passage in the Nicomachean Ethics:

> [I]f the acts that are in accordance with the excellences have themselves a certain character it does not follow that they are done justly or temperately. The agent also must be in a certain condition when he does them; in the first place he must have knowledge, secondly he must choose the acts, and choose them for their own sake, and thirdly his action must proceed from a firm and unchangeable character. (1105a 2–1105b 1)

The choice of what appears to be a virtuous act does not in itself guarantee that this act is in fact virtuous. A soldier may, for example, stand firm in the face of an enemy onslaught not because he is courageous, but rather because he is so overwhelmed with fear and terror that he cannot move! It is only a choice made in the context of a virtuous character which establishes an act as morally excellent. Actions may be called just and temperate when they are done as just and temperate persons do them.

Choice and practical wisdom are clearly key concepts in Aristotle's theory of moral virtue. So, finally, is the idea of training. Through the use of practical wisdom the moral agent is able to establish those passions and actions which over time are formative of character. It is in acting virtuously that a person eventually comes to possess this or that virtue. Just as a person becomes a lyre player by playing the lyre, one becomes just by doing just acts, brave by doing courageous acts, and so on (*NE* 1103a 31–1103b 1).

So what then is a virtue for Aristotle? It is 'a state concerned with choice, lying in a mean relative to us, this being determined by reason in the way in which the [person] of practical wisdom would determine it' (*NE* 1106b 36–1107a 1). In looking at Aquinas' theory, we will see most of these themes emerging, but they will be re-shaped through a theological orientation.

Aquinas on the virtues

Thomas Aquinas follows Aristotle in positing that the human, by nature, is orientated to a *telos*. However, he does something which his teacher was unable to do – namely, describe the role of the will in moving a person towards that goal. Further, while he agrees that happiness is the proximate end for the human person, he insists that her ultimate end is supernatural. The person who has the theological as well as the natural virtues is moving towards the ineffable glory of the beatific vision.

For Aquinas, there is one overarching, ultimate end to which the actions determined by will and reason is orientated. In his 'Commentary on Nichomachean Ethics', Aquinas (1988a) argues that where there are several goods identified, it is necessary to transcend the plurality in order to establish a superordinate end (I, lecture 9). There is a unity in human nature and it follows that the human person's ultimate end must be one. It is possible, some would say by way of objection, to construe the tendency to focus all one's actions on the one superordinate goal, even if it is a noble one, as distorted and unbalanced. This might be seen as somewhat obsessive or narrow. In order to overcome this problem, might it not be preferable to structure one's life around a series of interconnected goals? Porter (1990, p.78) has helpfully pointed out that Aquinas really intends something like this. The one end incorporates a number of different goods, pursued and enjoyed in a harmonious fashion. We can think of a superordinate goal and a number of subordinate goals. Thus, Aquinas (1969) can say that the human, if not directly seeking the perfect good, his ultimate end, is seeking a good 'as tending to that, for a start is made in order to come to a finish...' (*Summa Theologiae* I–II.1.6; *Summa* hereafter referred to as *ST*). A well-balanced person, for example, will have fun and recreation as one of her subordinate goals. She is aware that it is very difficult, if not impossible, to love God and neighbour fully if one's life is filled with duty and responsibility. One becomes stale, frustrated and bored. This is hardly the ground out of which a life of love and service is likely to spring.

Aquinas (1988b, 22.1.c) believes that every person naturally acts in such a way as to pursue what he perceives as the good. Clearly, it is possible for a person to be mistaken about what is good for him. But no one intentionally acts against the good. As McInerny (1993) expresses it:

> If we come to see that not-A rather than A contributes to our happiness, we have the same reason for doing not-A that we thought we had for doing A. We did A in the mistaken belief that it was good for us; when we learn that our judgment was mistaken, we do not need any further *reason* for not seeking A. We already and necessarily want what we think is good for us, and we now see that A is not. (pp.201–202)

To refer again to the example above, 'A' might be attempting to devote virtually all my free time to devotional activities and good works. The thinking is that in this way I will grow in holiness and experience a state of happiness that only the saints know. After a time, though, I find that rather than experiencing a new level of peace and joy, I simply end up feeling jaded. The saving grace comes when I discover the wisdom of 'not-A', achieving a balance in my life. I realise that in order to reach my superordinate goal of a deep union with God it is essential that I take a break to enjoy myself as well as devoting myself to serious Christian activity.

So the human person is essentially orientated to the good; she chooses acts which her reason tells her will move her towards the goal of happiness. Virtue, according to Aquinas (and following Aristotle), is that which makes the agent good and her acts also good (*ST* I–II.56.3). It is virtue, then, that disposes a person to act well, in accordance with her essential orientation to the end for which she was created. The question is, though, how does a person acquire virtue? Aquinas asks whether a virtuous disposition can be acquired through a single act (*ST* I–II.51.3). Clearly this is not possible. In order for virtue to become established in a person, reason must achieve mastery over 'the appetitive faculties' (our passions and desires). Now there is a whole range of situations involving a vast number of factors in which the desires come into play. It is not possible to establish right and good judgements in all these complex and diverse situations 'in an instant', so to speak. The virtuous disposition develops over time; it is a *habit*. It is a complicated business managing one's desires in order to establish virtue. A young business executive, for example, finds that there are a number of ways in which she can advance herself at the expense of others. She resists the temptation for a whole year and feels that she can now say that she has the virtue of justice. The problem is, though, that the temptation can surface in so many different forms. It is only through breadth of experience and through consistently choosing the right and good path that the virtue takes root. Aquinas would say, 'You've made a start, but you have not yet faced enough tempting situations to be able to say that the habit of justice is formed.' More formally, he puts it this way: 'The rational powers, proper to a [person], however, are not determined to one act, but rather in themselves are poised before many. It is through habits that they are set towards acts... Human virtues, therefore, are habits' (*ST* I–II.55.1).

As Hauerwas (1975, pp.69–70) points out, though, Aquinas' notion of a habit is quite different from our modern idea. We tend to think of a habit as something automatic, a rather mechanical function. One has, for example, the habit of each day buying a newspaper on the way home from work, reading it, and then walking the dog. For Aquinas, in contrast, a habit is a disposition to act well (or ill). So when he speaks of a virtue as a habit, he refers to a well-established disposition to act for the good. Habits are a 'readiness for action' (Hauerwas 1975, p.70).

We saw in our discussion of Aristotle's account of the virtues that his theory suffers through the lack of appreciation for the role of the *will* in relation to action. Aquinas, on the other hand, assigns the will a very important place in his moral psychology in general and in his theory of the virtues in particular. He says that the intellect is moved by the will, as all human faculties are (*ST* I–II.56.3). A person turns his mind in a certain direction because that is what he wants to do. The intellect, in this sense, is subordinate to the will. Thus, will is the subject of 'virtue in its unqualified sense' (*ST* I–II.56.3). The moral virtues are orientated to the will; the intellectual virtues to the rational powers.

> The subject of a habit which is called virtue in a certain respect can be the intellect [practical or speculative]... The subject of a habit which is

> downrightly called virtue, however, can only be the will… The reason for this is that the will moves to their acts all those other powers that are in some way rational… (*ST* I–II.56.3)

Put differently, it is a virtuous thing to use our rational powers to work on the various intellectual and practical challenges life throws up. But the moral life proper requires the exercise of the will. If we want to be persons of strong moral character, we need a consistent and strong intention to act for the good.

Aquinas, however, is not only interested in the way in which reason and appetite are well disposed in a person. His theological orientation leads him to ask how the supernatural virtues – faith, hope and love – are related to the natural virtues. It is not necessary for our purposes to describe how Aquinas understands the theological virtues. What we are interested in is how he construes the relationship between natural and supernatural virtues. (In the next chapter, the question of how a Christian presence might be distinguished from a natural presence will be pursued.)

Aquinas asks the question: 'Can the moral virtues exist without charity (a theological virtue)?' (*ST* I–II.65.2). In answering this question, he distinguishes between the proximate end for the human to which the moral virtues are orientated and the ultimate end attained through the theological virtues. The ultimate end for the human is that which she primarily desires. And the end of our desire is God.

> So the act by which we are primarily united to [God] is originally and essentially our happiness. But through the act of the intellect we are primarily united to him, and so the vision of God, which is an intellectual act, is essentially and originally our happiness. (Aquinas 1988c, 22.1.c)

While it is possible to acquire the moral virtues through human activity, and thus to move towards a temporal end, only those good deeds flowing from an infusion of God's love can direct a person to a supernatural last end. Thus, only the theological virtues ('infused' virtues) orientate a person to her ultimate end, and consequently they alone are perfect – virtues in an absolute sense. The moral virtues, with their orientation to the proximate end of (temporal) happiness, are virtues in a limited sense. While they may be considered true virtues, they are nonetheless incomplete.

In surveying the way Aristotle and Aquinas treat the virtues, we have noted some important differences. Aquinas assigns an important place to the role of the will in ordering the passions, and he places a supernatural *telos* above the proximate end of temporal happiness. A survey of other important virtue theorists would identify still more differences in emphasis and interpretation. Anyone interested in developing a system of virtue ethics is very quickly confronted with the question of whether or not it is possible to identify a unitary concept capable of tying together the vast array of interpretations. Alasdair MacIntyre sets himself this task in his influential and eloquent work *After Virtue* (MacIntyre 1985).

MacIntyre's notion of virtue and practices

MacIntyre, a moral theorist committed to the Aristotelian tradition, surveys accounts of virtue and the virtues from a wide variety of historical and cultural settings. Our aim here is simply to indicate just how diverse the various views on the virtues are. It is therefore not necessary to cover the full historical sweep contained in *After Virtue* (hereafter referred to as *AV*). A look at the key elements from the understanding of virtue in heroic societies and in the thought of Benjamin Franklin, taken together with what we have already seen of the teleological perspectives of Aristotle and Aquinas, will be sufficient to demonstrate plurality.

MacIntyre believes that in the concept of a practice it is possible to identify, at least in a partial sense, the place where much of the thinking on the virtues converges. Locating virtue within the context of practices, while offering a valuable perspective, is not adequate in itself. This move must be supplemented, according to MacIntyre, by setting the virtues in the perspective of the *telos* of a whole human life. The virtues should be understood not only as dispositions which sustain practices and the pursuit of the goods internal to them, but also as sustaining persons in their lifelong quest for the good.

MacIntyre observes that in a heroic society, such as that which was inspired by the epics of Homer, what is required of a person are actions (*AV*, ch.10): 'A man in heroic society is what he does' (*AV*, p.122). The virtues are those qualities which sustain a person in his role and which manifest themselves in the actions required by that role. The term *arete* is used for an excellence of any kind. A fast runner, for example, displays the *arete* of his feet. In a society where warfare played a dominant role, physical strength, courage and the skills of hand-to-hand combat would obviously all be virtues.

Morality and social structure are one and the same in heroic society. The particular moral structure shaping the society is represented in the heroic poetry (*AV*, pp.128–129). That structure has three central and interrelated elements. There is, first, the conception of what is required by the social role which each individual fulfils. Second, there is a conception of the excellences or virtues as those qualities which facilitate the carrying out of a role. Finally, we find a conception of the virtuous person as the one who, rather than trying to avoid vulnerability and death, gives them their due.

In a very different historical and cultural setting, Benjamin Franklin worked out his account of what it means to be virtuous (*AV*, pp.183, 185). He includes, notes MacIntyre, virtues one does not find in other lists namely, cleanliness, silence and industry. An acquisitive tendency, viewed by most of the ancient Greeks as the vice of *pleonexia*, is elevated to the status of a virtue. His view of chastity would sound very strange to earlier writers: 'Rarely use venery but for health or offspring – never to dullness, weakness or the injury of your own or another's peace or reputation' (Franklin; cited in *AV*, p.183).

While, observes MacIntyre, Franklin's account is, like Aristotle's, teleological, it differs significantly from the latter's in that it is also utilitarian. The aim of the virtuous life is happiness, but it is happiness understood as material success, a state of blessedness now, but also ultimately in heaven. The virtues are useful because they can move a person towards both material and spiritual happiness.

When we set these two conceptions of virtue and the virtues alongside the accounts developed by Aristotle and Aquinas, the differences are readily apparent and substantial. In Homeric society, a virtue is a quality which enables a person to fulfil his social role. Aristotle and Aquinas both view a virtue as moving a person towards his one end. Aquinas could agree that happiness in the temporal realm is a proximate end, but insists that the ultimate end is the perfect happiness of the beatific vision. Finally, for Franklin, a virtue is a quality which is useful in achieving temporal and eternal success.

MacIntyre sets himself the difficult task of endeavouring to find a unitary concept capable of tying these diverse views together. In doing this, he wants to stay within the parameters fixed by the Aristotelian tradition. He thinks that in a specially defined sense, the concept of a practice at least goes part way to achieving his aim. A practice is

> any coherent and complex form of socially established cooperative human activity through which goods internal to that form of activity are realized in the course of trying to achieve those standards of excellence which are appropriate to, and partially definitive of, that form of activity, with the result that human powers to achieve excellence, and human conceptions of the ends and goods involved, are systematically extended. (*AV*, p.187)

The parameters established by this definition are quite wide. Activities as diverse as fishing in a crew, architecture, sports, the arts and scientific endeavour all fit in. Given the wide net that is cast by the definition, a central question is this: How does one decide whether a human activity is in or out? Key words in the definition, such as 'complex' and 'cooperative', help us to identify those activities which do not fit in. While brick-laying involves skill, it is not a complex activity; one brick is laid on top of another over and over. It does not find a place. Basketball is a practice because it is co-operative, but the skill of shooting baskets (outside the context of a game) is not.

It is also important to note that in the definition there is an implicit contrast between goods *internal* to and goods *external* to a practice. There are some goods which are inherently associated with a practice. The very nature of the practice, the way it is constructed, determines those goods which are internal. MacIntyre (*AV*, p.188) uses the example of playing chess. Goods such as 'analytical skill' and 'strategic imagination' are established by the way the game itself is constructed. There are, however, goods which are externally associated with chess. One can gain wealth, fame and prestige by playing chess particularly well. But one may also attain these goods through activities completely unrelated to chess, such as acting, professional sport, and business.

Let me try to summarise the central ideas in MacIntyre's idea of a practice. In order to live well in this world of ours we need to co-operate with others in certain complex activities. From enjoying a game of chess or basketball, to constructing a multi-storey building, to working with others to promote health or education, people contribute their talents and abilities in order to achieve their collective goals. Now there are goods that are associated in a specific or inherent way with each of these activities. These are the goods or values that accrue because of the very nature of the activity required by this or that specific practice.

MacIntyre defines a virtue, in a partial and tentative way, in the context of the attainment of the goods inherent in practices: 'A virtue is an acquired human quality the possession and exercise of which tends to enable us to achieve those goods which are internal to practices and the lack of which effectively prevents us from achieving any such goods' (*AV*, p.191). In the context of chess, for instance, vision – the capacity to imaginatively project into the future – would be a virtue. Strategic imagination is a good internal to the practice of chess. In order to actualise this good, one needs to have vision.

As valuable as this approach to virtue is, there are, observes MacIntyre, obvious limitations. For example, there is in this scheme no way of resolving the potentially disastrous tensions arising out of conflicts in relation to the pursuit of different practices. A mother, for example, may be torn apart through conflict over raising her young children and pursuing her profession as an architect. The virtuous life needs a *telos* which transcends the limited goods of the practices and establishes the good of a whole human life (*AV*, p.203). The virtues, then, not only sustain practices and the pursuit of the goods internal to those practices, but also the lifelong quest for the good.

To recap, the notion of a practice is a preliminary, but nevertheless important, element in MacIntyre's interpretation of the virtuous life. In the next chapter, this concept will be used in developing the idea of presence as a virtue. It will be necessary to identify the way in which making oneself personally available functions in certain professional 'practices' to actualise the goods inherent in those practices. It is natural to look to the hospital, the psychotherapist's office and the school to find places where presence is a virtue. The practices we will analyse will be nursing, midwifery, psychotherapy and teaching.

CHAPTER 3

Self-Communication as a Virtue in the Human Service Professions

The aim in this chapter is to develop the notion that there are certain professional practices in which self-communication is a virtue. The professional practices to be analysed are nursing care, midwifery, education and psychotherapy. An attempt will be made to show how in each one self-gifting contributes significantly to the attainment of the goods internal to it. Clearly, professional skills are important in all of these practices. I will be suggesting, however, that these skills need to be combined with personal availability if the goals in the endeavour are to be optimally realised. We will discover that in the literature associated with the four professions, a large number of terms are used to express the idea of being available. To give of the self in service of the other involves warmth, caring and support. It entails empathy, presence and attunement. It is about, finally, encouragement, affirmation and respect. Or in Marcelian language, it is about an act of belonging. For a time, one is prepared to substitute the needs of the other for one's own. In the human service professions, I will be arguing, this offering of self is a virtue.

Self-communication is obviously a quality which is central in the Christian life. Indeed, to make oneself available to another person is an expression of *agape*. Christ commanded us to love our neighbours. If we love our neighbours we will be prepared to give of ourselves in the interests of their psychological and spiritual well-being. Christians working in service professions will want to develop their capacity for self-communication. But Christians do not, of course, have a monopoly on either love or self-communication. If self-gifting has both a natural and a Christian application, it seems important to ask how, if at all, the two differ. Is it the case, for example, as Aquinas would argue, that the person who makes himself disposable for others without an infusion of divine love manifests only *incomplete* virtue? Is natural self-communication somehow inferior to Christian self-communication? It will be argued that the two should not be distinguished in terms of perfection (or imperfection), but rather with reference to *vision*. That is to say, a Christian has a particular vision of herself, of life, of the other, of God. It is a vision formed out of the key metaphors and images in the Christian story. The fact, for example, that a Christian trains herself to see Christ in the other will, or should, have a profound effect on her mode of self-communication. This notion of the link between vision and availability will be developed. We will begin, however, with an analysis of the moral dimension of self-communication in the people-orientated professions.

Self-communication as a virtue in personal service practices

What is central in MacIntyre's notion of a practice is that it indicates a co-operative endeavour in which certain human powers are exercised to maximise the realisation of the goods internal to that endeavour. That is, when persons engage in a particular activity through co-ordinating their skills, talents and energies in pursuit of the goods associated with that activity, they are involved in a practice. Below we will discuss four human service practices: nursing care, midwifery, education and psychotherapy. The process will be to identify the goods internal to the particular practice, and then to demonstrate that self-communication is a capacity in the professional which contributes significantly to the attainment of those goods. In all cases, professional skills play a very important role. To assist a person's recovery from ill-health, a nurse needs to be clinically competent. Midwives, similarly, need the technical skills to competently assist in routine births and to deal effectively with minor complications. Teachers need to be proficient in educational process if they are to assist students in actualising their learning potential. And finally, skills and techniques play an important role in all forms of therapy. What I will be arguing, however, is that all of these practices require of their practitioners a capacity for self-communication if the goods are to be optimally attained. The ideal is a practitioner who is technically competent and personally available. Without the capacity of self-gifting, it is not possible to attain the goal of excellence, which is a central element in MacIntyre's definition of a practice. In human service practices, I will be arguing, self-communication is a virtue.

As we review the scholarly literature on relationality in personal service, we will encounter words such as 'presence', 'affirmation', 'empathy', 'attunement' and 'respectfulness'. In a Marcelian framework, this word group refers to belonging. When I commit myself to belong to another, I am committing myself to a donation of my personal resources for the sake of her needs. Marcel says that this involves a substitution of freedom. I substitute her freedom for my own. But this does not mean that a commitment to belonging ends in being reduced to slave status. In the paradoxical terms of the gospel, to lose oneself for the sake of another and for the sake of the gospel is to find oneself. To substitute freedom in an act of service is to be free in the deepest sense. The nurse, the midwife, the teacher or the counsellor who is prepared to communicate self in helping the other establishes the experience of belonging. When there is availability, attunement, encouragement and respect the service provider and the other feel that they belong together. To be able to establish a sense of belonging with another is a virtue.

Nursing care

The central good associated with a stay in hospital is a return to full health. The patient and the medical staff work together with the aim of ensuring that the recovery is speedy and optimally comfortable. While the primary quality required to achieve these goods is clinical competence, a caring presence has traditionally been valued in nursing. Nursing care is generally acknowledged to have a holistic concern. It is recognised that the patient has spiritual and emotional as well as physical needs. To take the case of recovery from a major surgical procedure, the patient is in a highly vulnerable and dependent situation. During the early stages of recovery the pain is obviously intense, perhaps almost overwhelming. While the capacity to deliver effective pain relief is what the patient will value most highly, the compassionate presence of the nurse is also prized. In the extremity of his situation, the smallest offering of concern and care may assume mammoth proportions. Even if the patient is quite groggy and not fully aware of what is taking place around him, the dim recognition of a benevolent presence is sufficient to engender a feeling of security. The fact that she has been able to offer herself in caring and concern means that the nurse has included herself in the pain, anxiety and disorientation of her patient. While maintaining her position as nurse, she has gone over to the other side in her imagination to experience something of what it is to be a patient. More precisely, she has entered into the experience of this particular patient – the one she is currently with. If all that she were in contact with were her thoughts and feelings as a nurse, she would be cut off from her patient and there would be no possibility of her meeting him as a compassionate presence.

While the primary concern of patient and nurse alike is likely to be the nurse's technical competence, the overall quality of the recuperative process will be judged by the patient not only in terms of the technical skill of the nursing, but also in terms of the level of compassion and self-giving in the nursing presence. It is quite misguided to suggest that it really does not matter a great deal whether or not a nurse attempts to create a supportive environment, that the essential thing is her technical skill. Quite apart from the fact that a positive psychological and emotional state may well aid physical recovery, patients consistently report their deep appreciation for the compassionate presence of the nursing staff.

In describing the compassionate presence of the nurse, the pastoral theologian Alastair Campbell helpfully develops the images of *mothering* and *skilled companionship* (Campbell 1984, pp.41–42, 49–51). 'The "nurse as mother",' he writes, 'is a warm presence in a frightening world, just as the real mother's cuddling soothes away her baby's fears… The body, which has become a source of such discomfort and fear, is handled both competently and lovingly' (Campbell 1984, pp.41–42).

However, there are problems, observes Campbell, with this model of nursing. Nurses, first, are not in fact mothers, and tender care is not a peculiarly feminine trait. Second, if a nurse thinks of herself as a mother she may tend to foster dependency in the patient, thus failing to encourage him to take appropriate responsibility for his own recuperation. For these reasons, Campbell prefers the image of the companion. This image has the advantages of pointing to a closeness which, on the one hand, avoids gender stereotypes and, on the other, expresses mutuality. Companionship 'describes a closeness which is neither sexual union nor deep personal friendship. It is a bodily presence which accompanies the other for a while' (Campbell 1984, p.49).

Interestingly, some nursing scholars argue that beyond the good of a companioned recovery there is the good of the patient gaining intellectual and interpersonal competencies. Underlining the thought of the American nursing theorist Hildegard Peplau, Gastmans (1998) contends that nursing practice is educative and growth promoting. The nurse aims to promote in the patient an increase in her capacity for constructive and creative engagement with others. In such a view, relationality is at the heart of nursing practice:

> [B]oth the patient and the nurse contribute to and participate in promoting the relational process which unfolds between them. The nurse and the patient are conceived as human persons, each with their own fields of experience and perception, constituted by thoughts, feelings, desires, assumptions, expectations and activities. The interaction between the thoughts, feelings and activities of the patient and those of the nurse lies at the very centre of the nursing process. (Gastmans 1998, pp.1315–1316)

Here Buber, I suggest, has an important contribution to make. The interaction between the two personal 'fields' is founded on an act of inclusion. It is only when one becomes aware of the 'field of experience and perception' of the other that one can engage in genuine communication. It is through 'swinging' into the inner world of the patient that the nurse is able to establish his emotional and spiritual needs and to attempt to meet them.

Gwen Hartrick joins Gastmans in according relationality a central place. She refers to it as 'the foundation of nursing practice' (Hartrick 1997, p.526). In order to contribute maximally to people's health and healing experiences nurses need a highly developed 'relational capacity'. Hartrick (1997) contends that interpersonal virtuosity is not achieved simply through the acquisition of a set of 'behavioral communication skills' (e.g. empathy, self-disclosure, clarifying and confronting) but through a capacity 'to relate in a spontaneously human manner' (p.524; her emphasis). (I am not altogether comfortable with the notion of empathy as a 'behavioral communication skill'. To think and feel oneself into the inner world of experience of the other involves more than communication skills. It requires personal availability.) The problem with a 'mechanistic' approach, one which emphasises behavioural communication skills, Hartrick observes, is that it tends to induce self-consciousness and a focus on technical correctness. Relational connectedness requires self-abandonment, and self-consciousness mitigates the capacity to let go of self.

> When a nurse has the initiative to be with another in an authentic way, she or he is able to respond to the other, expressing the feelings she or he has as they emerge. There is no struggle to look for 'the right thing to say', but rather the focus is on being with another person, listening to one's experiencing of the other, and responding to the other by expressing the feelings and thoughts that emerge. (Hartrick 1997, p.526)

Within nursing scholarship now there are those who advocate moving past the clinical/technological paradigm to one which emphasises person-to-person caring. In the new paradigm, the nurse has a holistic concern, even daring to hold as an aim the psychological and spiritual maturing of the person in and through the process of recovery. To achieve this aim, the nurse needs to enhance her or his capacity for authenticity, responsiveness, mutuality and self-abandonment.

Midwifery

In seeking to identify the goods associated with childbirth, one must look to the experience of women. Two primary goods they nominate are *fulfilment/satisfaction* and *control* (Green, Coupland and Kitzinger 1990). The sense of fulfilment/satisfaction a woman feels in the birthing experience is associated with a number of factors. These include the following: the degree of difficulty of the delivery, the nature of interventions, the use of pain relief, the quality of staff care, and the level of participation in and control over the birth process (Green *et al.* 1990, p.18). Given the inclusion of the last mentioned factor in the list, it is evident that the two goods are closely linked. Control is a term which has two referents, namely self-control and control over the management of the labour. With regard to both these dimensions of control there is ambiguity (Green *et al.* 1990, p.16). While some theorists, first, emphasise the importance of the woman maintaining control over her behaviour (through the use of relaxation techniques, for example), others suggest that a positive childbirth experience requires following the lead given by one's body rather than being concerned with control. With reference to a sense of control over decision making and clinical actions, some professionals argue that allowing women to become too involved in these processes is not so much empowering as confusing and anxiety producing. There is, however, strong empirical evidence indicating that women who do not feel in control in the childbirth process – in control either of themselves or of their environment – feel dissatisfied and lack a sense of fulfilment (Green *et al.* 1990, p.21).

In attempting to help women secure these goods, the midwife needs to be both clinically competent and therapeutically available. As Kitzinger (1988) observes, to pit the model of the midwife which emphasises warmth, wisdom and caring against the model highlighting the importance of clinical competence is to set up a false dichotomy:

> For the midwife cannot be skilled without being caring. She cannot be truly caring without being skilled. All those who work with childbearing women owe it to them to develop skills and knowledge, and to question all received opinion... It is also the responsibility of every one of us to examine critically *all* dogmas...to ask for the evidence and investigate the benefits and hazards of such things as shaving of the perineum, enemas and suppositories, putting women to bed in labour, routine intravenous infusions, commanded pushing and prolonged breath-holding in the second stage, routine episiotomy, and every one of the rules and regulations and customary practices in hospitals today. (pp.7–8)

Clinical skills and relational capacity are indissolubly linked in the quest to secure the goods associated with the practice of childbirth. It is the second factor that we are concentrating on here. We are searching for an answer to the question: What are the qualities in the midwife which contribute to the goal of a satisfying and fulfilling labour and delivery? In reviewing the midwifery literature, I have discovered four such qualities, namely *authentic communication, presence, attunement* and *respectfulness*.

Rogers (1990a) posited genuineness or congruence as one of the hallmarks of an authentic therapeutic relationship. In order to be trustworthy with the other, it is not that one has to be absolutely consistent (an impossible ideal), but rather 'dependably real'. To be 'real' or genuine in a relationship, it is necessary to get in touch with one's feelings and to *be* those feelings with the other. Midwifery scholars also refer to the importance of *authentic communication*: 'Midwives who are in touch with their own being,' writes Siddiqui (1999), 'are their own source, and can be a source to others for whom they are caring and teaching. The authentic encounter in midwifery is founded upon the midwife who is a personal source and who can be a therapeutic source from self to others' (p.112).

Presence refers to the capacity to bring one's self to bear positively on a relationship. When a person makes her presence felt the other experiences an increase in her sense of well-being. It is vitally important in midwifery. 'The element of presence is both complex and simple, and relates to the midwife in contact with the woman who is the centre of the relationship' (Siddiqui 1999, p.112). A common expression of a defective presence by staff during labour is engaging in social banter (Siddiqui 1999). While some will seek to justify this practice on the basis of it serving to relieve tension, it is likely that the woman will construe it as a failure to acknowledge the significance of her experience. In this case, she will feel alienated from her attendants. This observation highlights the importance of the midwife being *attuned* to the childbirth experience.

'Understanding and interpreting what the woman is experiencing is at the core of midwifery care...' (Robinson 1997, p.45). Attunement is another word for inclusion. The midwife imaginatively goes over into the experience of the woman. A central experience for a labouring woman is that of 'going into herself'. For a time, the woman cuts herself off from our world and does a sort of 'inner trip' (Odent 1996, p.304). One woman described the experience as a 'hiding in the self': 'You go into yourself, I don't know how to explain it, but hide in yourself, and that you know that this is going to end' (Lungren and Dahlberg 1998, p.107). In reflecting on this experience, Odent (1996) makes this important comment:

> Birth attendants who have understood this essential aspect of the physiology of labor and delivery avoid any unnecessary neocortical stimulation [the neocortical structures of the brain are associated with inhibitions] that can interfere with the progress of the labor. They will be cautious not to talk unnecessarily, and refrain from using a 'rational' language. (pp.304–305)

Odent presents an extraordinary woman, Gisèle, as an exemplar of an attuned, non-intrusive presence. She was educated as a midwife in the 1940s.

> When Gisèle looked after a laboring woman, one could often find this typical scenario: no one was in the small, dimly lighted room other than the mother to be and Gisèle, who sat in a corner, knitting. She could spend

hours and hours knitting. Her technique and speed were impressive! And it was usually unremarkable when a first baby was born in three or four hours.

In a very small number of cases, not exceeding 2% of the births, Gisèle was in a position to decide that a technique other than silent knitting was needed. (Odent 1996, p.304)

Obviously the point is not that contemporary midwives should take over Gisèle's technique. Rather, her style is important for at least two reasons. First, she points to the importance of 'mothering' in the childbirth experience. Gisèle takes us back to the roots of midwifery. In days gone by the midwife was essentially a mother figure. She provided a sense of security and protection during an extremely demanding and scary experience. And second, Gisèle manifests an instinctive, intuitive attunement to the birthing process. In a remarkable way, she set herself at a slight distance from the labouring woman and yet at the same time was able to communicate a total involvement in the woman's experience.

Being fully present, attuned, involved – these are the behaviours that communicate *respect* to the woman. Apart from the midwife's personal presence, her mediation of the physical aspects of the therapeutic relationship is of prime importance in manifesting her basic respect for the woman in her care. Flint (1995) refers, for example, to the physical position of women throughout antenatal and intrapartum care. In most obstetric units, that position is horizontal. 'It is difficult,' she observes, 'for even the most articulate woman to think rationally, discuss, negotiate and inquire in such a disadvantageous position… Horizontal women do not feel in control of their situation and it is not helpful to their concepts of their own value and self-worth' (p.19).

In reflecting further on the meaning of respect and dignity during labour and delivery, Flint (1995, p.25) refers to a birth, of baby Joanna, in which the mother delivered on all fours, completely naked, with her bottom in the air ('for 45 minutes during the labour I never saw the mother's face'). After the labour the mother looked at Flint 'with shining eyes' and said: 'Thank you, Caroline, that was so lovely, so dignified. I really felt in control of the whole thing.' Flint found herself comparing Joanna's birth to the mother's first. It was very different. In her first experience, she had had an induction, an epidural, and she had been electronically monitored throughout. She had optimal pain relief from the epidural, laboured on a bed, and had kept her clothes on throughout.

> In theory, that labour sounds as if it were much more dignified than this one; dressed instead of naked, no pain so no grunts, no groans or sounds of pushing, a covered woman sitting on a bed instead of a naked woman with no face, and yet Joanna's mother was ecstatic about the delivery and labour this time.

Flint concludes that according the woman respect and facilitating a labour and delivery of dignity is not about keeping gowns on and sedating, it is not even ultimately about providing optimal pain relief, but rather is associated with handing the labour over to the woman and 'keep[ing] a low-profile'. Perhaps it is about offering a presence that lives in the tension of distance and closeness, of quietness and intensity, and of letting be and confronting.

Skills and scientific knowledge are clearly very important in the practice of midwifery. But it is only when the midwife provides a wise and befriending presence that the woman is able, with Joanna's mother, to say, 'Thank you. That was so lovely, so dignified.'

Education

The term *education* has, of course, a very wide application. I want here to concentrate on the education of adolescents, although reference will be made at one point to younger children. A primary good in the practice of classroom education is optimal engagement by students with the learning process. A high level of motivation is important both for the significant contribution it makes to academic achievement, and for the lifelong pattern of commitment to personal and professional development that it establishes. Student engagement has both behavioural and affective dimensions (Skinner and Belmont 1993). Motivated students attempt tasks which require an extension of present capacities and understanding, show high levels of persistence in the face of difficulties, and take the initiative when given the opportunity. They also display positive emotions such as interest, enthusiasm and curiosity.

We need to ask: What model or models of the educational process encourage students to fully engage with their studies? Bruner (1996) presents three contemporary approaches to learning in advanced societies (his first model, 'children as imitative learners', relates to traditional societies): the didactic, intersubjective and the interpretive retrieval approaches.[1]

The first approach is the one that we are perhaps most familiar with. The teacher sets about informing her pupils of certain facts, principles and rules. The aim is for students to learn, remember and then apply the information. What is to be learned resides in the mind of the teacher, as well as in books, maps and computer databases. There is an obvious need for students to build up a store of factual knowledge. This approach certainly has a place in modern education. Its weakness, however, lies in its basic assumption – namely, that the child's mind is passive and active interpretation is unnecessary. 'The didactic bias views the child from the outside, from a third-person perspective, rather than trying to "enter her thoughts". It is blankly one-way: teaching is not a mutual dialogue, but a telling by one to the other' (Bruner 1996, p.56). It is difficult to see how a teacher would fully engage her pupils if the didactic bias were strong in her educational philosophy. What Bruner calls 'a first-person perspective', an attempt to think oneself into the inner domain of the child (Buber's notion of inclusion), is required if the teacher is to foster a love of learning. It is this first-person perspective which is central in the intersubjective approach.

In a 'pedagogy of mutuality' the child's perspective is recognised and valued. There is an understanding that children, like adults, construct a model of the world in helping them interpret their experience. In a project of learning grounded in intersubjectivity, the first step is to imaginatively grasp the child's model of reality. Then it is possible to introduce other perspectives in order to expand and develop the child's intellectual constructs. Importantly, these alternative views are not imposed on the student. That she is capable of reasoning, interpretation and evaluation is fully acknowledged. In this approach, knowledge and truth are not seen as entities that are transmitted from the active mind of the teacher to the passive mind of the pupil. Rather, learning is set in the context of mutuality. On these matters, Bruner (1996) is eloquent:

> Knowledge is what is shared within discourse, within a 'textual' community. Truths are the product of evidence, argument, and construction rather than of authority, textual or pedagogic. This model of education is mutualist and dialectical, more concerned with interpretation

and understanding than with the achievement of factual knowledge or skilled performance. (p.62)

The third approach combines elements of the first two. There is a tradition of knowledge and learning that is objectively 'there'. In her educational development the student must engage with that tradition. Along with one's own ideas on how to construct a literary work, one is also confronted by those of Shakespeare, Dostoevsky and Tolkien. Education is not simply a process of developing personal, idiosyncratic views. It involves questioning and learning from the great tradition of scholarship. 'Those presently engaged in the pursuit of knowledge become sharers in conjectures with those long dead' (Bruner 1996, p.62). In sharing in the quest for understanding and wisdom with their intellectual ancestors, students cannot simply borrow the perspectives of those ancestors – they must retrieve them for the contemporary world through a process of interpretation and contextualisation.

I contend that when the capacities and values of the student are acknowledged (a 'first-person perspective'), when learning is viewed as shared praxis (a 'pedagogy of mutuality'), and when interpretive engagement with the tradition is encouraged (sharing in 'the conjectures of those long dead'), the potential for enhancing student motivation is high. In order to facilitate this approach to education, a teacher needs certain skills and, more importantly from our point of view, she needs to be personally available to her pupils. Let us consider, first, some of the fundamental skills that are required (on this, see Brophy 1986). The teacher must, for example, be able to adapt curriculum materials to meet the particular needs of her students. She must be able, also, to pace the learning process appropriately. In order to help pupils develop their models of the world, it is necessary for the teacher to help them to make connections between existing and new knowledge. If the process is carried along too rapidly, students will be unable to make the connections and will become discouraged. Questioning of students, finally, is an important element in shared learning praxis. Effective teachers understand how to appropriately mix those questions focused on facts and information with those orientated to comprehension and interpretation. Moreover, they understand how to appropriately sequence the questions and how to follow up responses to build the scaffold of learning. And there are, of course, many other skills that could be listed. Our focus, however, is not on teacher technique but on teacher availability. The aim is to identify the ways in which the teacher needs to extend herself personally in order to heighten learner engagement.

In analysing the operation of the collaborative school culture advocated by Bruner, it is evident, I suggest, that a teacher needs to make herself personally available to students in three crucial ways. First, she needs to include herself in the child's way of constructing his model of the world. Second, she needs to offer support, affirmation and encouragement during the risky and challenging work of interpretation and dialogue. And finally, she needs to facilitate the building of the collaborative learning community.

Adopting a 'first-person perspective' in the classroom means, in Buberian terms, including oneself in the experience of the learner. The teacher imaginatively swings into the inner domain of the pupil. This is an activity which requires her to extend herself. Not only is it necessary for her to call upon her powers of imagination, she must also exercise patience. She must engage in a process of checking interpretations against feedback from the student until a relatively close match is achieved. It is necessary for her to persevere in order to understand. In expending mental energy and in exercising patience the teacher makes herself available to her pupils.

Seeing the learning process as the child does is a necessary first step. In order to move the process forward through engaging in a dialogue with him, it is necessary to establish a supportive learning environment. Arguing one's case, responding to challenges, and engaging with the great thinkers and writers in the intellectual tradition are activities which require a relatively high level of self-confidence. There are now a number of empirical studies which indicate that in order to help students engage fully with these learning processes it is necessary for the teacher to provide emotional support and encouragement. Under the rubric of 'involvement', Skinner and Belmont (1993) refer to teachers who 'take time for, express affection toward, enjoy interactions with, are attuned to, and dedicate resources to their students' (p.573). They found that teacher involvement has a significant impact not only on students' feelings of belonging but also on their sense of competence and autonomy. In their study of the relationship between the psychological environment in lower secondary school classrooms and motivation, Roeser, Midgley and Urdan (1996) incorporated both academic and relational factors. With respect to the latter, they observed that teachers who show respect and care and who provide encouragement help generate a sense of belonging. When students feel that they belong, the authors discovered, their self-esteem and learning confidence are boosted and, as a result, their self-consciousness in learning situations is mitigated. In their research, Cooper and McIntyre (1996) confirm these findings. Understanding education as a 'transactional' process involving communication and co-operation means, they say, that the affective dimension is of great significance. The pupil needs a positive sense of self-worth and a strong sense of academic efficacy.

> This requires an emotionally supportive environment, in which the learner feels valued and respected by significant others (i.e. teachers and fellow pupils) with whom he or she is expected to interact in the learning process. (Cooper and McIntyre 1996, p.97)

It is worth repeating here an extract from the research by Cooper and McIntyre (1996) which illustrates vividly the important role of the teacher in affirmation and encouragement. One of the classes observed by the researchers was studying the difference between 'Standard English' and 'dialect'. In endeavouring to come to grips with the concepts, a pupil, Jim, thought of a trunk and branch metaphor: 'There's just one stalk with the dialects branching off. And if they want to make a new word, they come back to the branch and out sprouts another twig' (p.101). In commenting on his response to Jim's suggestive image, the teacher reveals a propensity for self-communication in the educational process:

> I think Jim is a good example of that [he is referring to matching subjective understandings] because normally I think he's perhaps very frustrated by his perceived levels of achievement, because, as we said before, he has problems with his writing... So just that one lesson where he came out with that wonderful example that I told you about before [i.e. the tree analogy], when I took that out and said, 'Right! I'm going to use that now. That's so good! I'm going to use that in future because that's really sharpened my thinking.' And because I made a big fuss over that, and particularly stressed it in the lesson – kept going on about it, and I kept using it in front of the class – you know, I could visibly see him perk up and start to puff his chest out a bit and engage more in the lesson... And all the way through the rest of the work his oral contribution was far

more significant [than usual] because, I think, he felt a bit more ownership. And I wrote it on the board, and some of them put it in their books... And he could see his idea going down into people's books. (pp.101–102)

The teacher had clearly entered into Jim's customary experience of frustration in the learning process. That he is now genuinely excited that his pupil has had this flash of inspiration is obvious. The teacher is really pleased for Jim. Moreover, he cares enough to make the most of the situation in enhancing Jim's self-esteem and self-confidence.

The teacher is here modelling the kind of supportive, encouraging learning community that is required to facilitate education which is focused not simply on passively receiving information but on actively constructing meanings. It is risky to try out one's ideas on a new subject. In such a situation, one looks for understanding and support not only from the teacher, but also from one's co-learners. The teacher needs to engage personally in the process of building a collaborative learning community through modelling appropriate attitudes and behaviours. Moreover, she needs to take the time and expend the effort to correct actions which mitigate self-confidence and self-esteem in others. In this way, the ethos of the learning community will develop over time as one which is characterised by supportiveness, encouragement, respect and mutuality. Bruner (1996) finds in a school in Oakland, California, an exemplar of this kind of collaborative community:

When I visited the school, the [lower primary] students were studying the aftermath of the *Exxon Valdez* oil spill in Alaska. Their aim was to come up with a Plan. And in the interest of the Plan they were willing to entertain all possible proposals, however 'wild,' knowing that others would listen and nobody would make fun of their ideas. One of the 'hot ideas' during the visit, for example, was that you could get oil off birds using peanut butter as an 'oil blotter.' There was no mocking about it: they pushed the idea to the limits, arguing that peanut butter should be easy to get since 'there's so much of it anyway.' These children had learned to treat ideas respectfully, pragmatically, and actively. They were seriously engaged in trying to justify to a problem-solving community why 'oil blotters' might be a great idea for rescuing birds caught in an oil spill, and in doing so they were 'teaching' each other in the egalitarian sense – and, indeed, were part of a community whose aim was just such 'teaching by sharing.' (pp.76–77)

In shaping a collaborative community of learning such as this, the teacher needs to bring something more than skills and techniques. It is her personal input, her self-communication, which encourages respect and supportiveness on the one hand, and risk taking, creativity and a love of ideas on the other.

Psychotherapy

The last practice to be considered, psychotherapy, is one in which most laypersons would expect self-communication to be a prominent feature. Certainly there are a number of schools of psychotherapy in which this is the case. But not all schools elevate the role of presence and compassion. The aim here is to identify approaches in which self-communication is viewed as the most potent resource available to the therapist in promoting healing and growth.

The goods of therapy are variously described. If asked, clinicians would refer to one or more of the following: a lowering in levels of anxiety, mood elevation, an enhanced ego strength, a greater level of personal autonomy, an enhanced capacity for rational engagement with life, and the emergence of the real or organismic self. While there is in all schools of therapy an appreciation of the importance of empathy and acceptance, the amount of weight assigned to the relational qualities of the therapist in achieving therapeutic goals varies. In some schools there is a greater emphasis on skills and techniques than on the meeting between the therapist and the client. A significant number of therapists interpret their role primarily in terms of technical skills such as the interpretation of dream material (psychoanalysis), reframing (brief therapy), and reshaping distorted patterns of thought (cognitive therapy).

Perhaps in classical psychoanalysis we find the approach to therapy in which the relational dimension is accorded the least value. In Freud's view, the analyst takes on the role of a detached, analytical observer. He operates in a state of 'evenly hovering attention', attempting all the while to formulate the dynamics associated with the intrapsychic conflict in the patient. In probing the unconscious, the analyst must deal with the thwarting capability of resistances. Free association provides a means of bypassing these defence mechanisms. As the material from the unconscious becomes available, the analyst needs to clear her presuppositions in order to accurately formulate the intrapsychic dynamics. The analyst is present in the role of a detached, quasi-scientific observer. Her primary aim is to reach that point of objective understanding of the intrapsychic conflict which indicates how she should intervene to bring the patient to insight and cure. We must be careful, however, not to under-estimate the role of the relational in psychoanalytic therapy. A central place in the treatment of neurosis is accorded to transference. Transference refers to a phenomenon in which the client begins to relate to the therapist as if she were a significant figure, usually a parent, in his personal history. It is when the neurosis is mobilised through an activation of early conflicts and traumas within the therapeutic relationship that healing really begins. What is important in the context of our present discussion is that transference is a relational phenomenon.

Even though in all approaches to therapy there is an acknowledgement that the relationship between the therapist and the client is important, there is an emerging 'school' in which being fully present and available is identified as the critical factor in achieving therapeutic goals. The existentialist therapist Irvin Yalom tells a story which illustrates well the convictions of the members of this school (Yalom 1980, pp.1–2). As a student, he went with a group of his friends to visit an old Armenian lady to learn the art of producing fine cuisine. Yalom would assiduously follow her recipes, but he could never reproduce the wonderful taste sensations he experienced at the home of his tutor. One evening, while waiting at her table to receive his meal, he noticed that as the young female servant brought the food to the table, she quickly and as inconspicuously as possible threw in a range of condiments. There was the answer to the puzzle! The extra touch he was missing out on came from what the servant girl added in between the kitchen and the table. He offers this experience as a psychotherapeutic parable. While, he observes, the psychotherapeutic profession likes to attribute its successes to highly technical factors such as strategic interventions, the development and resolution of transference, and the analysis of object relations, 'when no one is looking, the therapist throws in the "real thing"' (Yalom 1980, p.3). It is easy to list but difficult to define the 'extras' which contribute so substantially to client improvement. Included in this collection of therapeutic qualities are the following:

'compassion, "presence", caring, extending oneself, touching the patient at a profound level...[and] wisdom' (Yalom 1980, p.4).

What Yalom presents here is a conviction which unites a group of theorists and clinicians with various psychotherapeutic pedigrees into a loose school of thought which I would term 'relational therapy'.[2] Carl Rogers was a pioneer in this 'school'. He argued that the way the therapist is present to the client is the really critical factor in therapy. In his understanding of what constitutes genuine presence in the therapeutic relationship, he was significantly influenced by Martin Buber, referring to him as one of his favourite thinkers (Rogers 1980, p.41). Rogers (1969, p.232) described the experience in therapy of a 'deep realness in one [meeting] a deep realness in the other' as an I–Thou moment. He identified three key attitudes in the project of establishing a healing relationship, namely acceptance, genuineness (or congruence) and empathy (Rogers 1990b). It is absolutely essential, he contended, that the therapist communicate acceptance or unconditional positive regard to the client. She, the client, must know that everything she is feeling – aggression, anger, guilt and lust along with more positive affects – is accepted by the therapist. This accepting, 'prizing' attitude provides the client with a unique opportunity to really understand herself.

Acceptance, however, must not be confused with 'phoniness'. In order for the therapist to establish himself as trustworthy, he must be 'dependably real'. 'Genuineness means that the therapist is openly being the feelings and attitudes flowing within at the moment' (Rogers 1990b, p.135). There must be, in other words, a congruence between what he is presently feeling at 'gut level' and what he expresses to the client.

Empathy, lastly, is the capacity to think and feel oneself into the inner world of the client. Imaginatively, the therapist is able to begin, at least, to see the feelings and personal meanings as the client does. Rogers (1990b, p.136) held that the therapist who is sensitive and attuned could even grasp meanings just outside the client's awareness.

With an orientation to helping persons engage honestly with their potentialities, to experience their existence as fully as possible, it is to be expected that at least some existentialist therapists would also find a place here. Alongside Yalom, we find Rollo May (1983), James Bugental (1987) and Jim Lantz (1994a, 1994b). In order to get the flavour of this approach, I will highlight key features in the approaches of May and Bugental.

May (1983) characterises therapy in terms of an encounter between therapist and client aimed at helping the latter '*experience his existence as real*' (p.156; his emphasis). For her part, the therapist needs to be fully 'present'. That is, she needs to facilitate a 'total relationship', one which operates on a number of levels (May 1983, p.21). The levels include 'realness', friendship, *agape* and *eros*.

Bugental (1987) also identifies the 'presence' of both therapist and client as the heart of therapy:

> Looking back now, it is surprising to me how long I overlooked the fundamental importance of presence to therapeutic work. It is even more surprising to me how many therapists and therapeutic systems also overlook it. All too often, therapists seem to be so attentive to the content of what is being said and to their prior conceptions about client dynamics and needs that they don't notice the distance that exists between themselves and their partners. (p.46)

The art of therapy consists of reducing that distance to the point where there is a real meeting, a sharing in presence. 'Accessibility' and 'expressiveness' in the client are indicators that she is really present in the therapeutic relationship (Bugental 1987, p.27). The former term refers to openness to the 'press' for change and growth coming from the therapist; whereas the latter identifies a genuine, honest sharing of subjective experience.

Another important figure in this school is the British psychotherapist Robert Hobson. He takes an eclectic approach to therapy; however, his background is Jungian. The stress he places on relationship in therapy is evident in the name he gives to his approach, namely the *Conversational Model*. Therapist and client, alone and together, develop a 'feeling-language':

> *Dialogue* entails the recognition of the other person as an experiencing subject. In a simultaneous acting and being acted upon, knowing and being known, there is a mutual creation of a personal feeling-language. 'I and you' becomes 'I–Thou'. Empathy, a one-way apprehension of what Joe Bloggs is experiencing, moves towards a mutual understanding in which Joe and I are at once alone and together. (Hobson 1985, p.194)

According to Hobson, healing begins when the client is able to share those images of pain, anxiety and alienation which arise in the heart. It is the therapist's dialogic presence, creating with the client a mutuality that encompasses both individuality and communion (aloneness–togetherness), which facilitates this movement into 'feeling-images'.

In the psychoanalytic tradition, mention could be made of Kohut's (1971, 1977, 1984) self-psychology and the research into the place of empathic presence in psychoanalysis by Stolorow, Brandchaft and Atwood (1987). In the 1960s and 1970s Kohut established himself as a leading theorist and practitioner in the treatment of narcissistic personality disorder. The narcissistic personality, according to Kohut (1977, p.5), suffers from feelings of emptiness and depression, of inferiority and rejection, and of not being fully real. Based on his clinical experience, he contends that what these depleted selves need most is to admire (to 'idealise') and to be admired ('mirrored').

The disorder can be traced, he holds, to large-scale empathic failures on the part of parents (they reject the child's attempts at idealisation or they fail to mirror adequately). In therapy, Kohut stresses empathy and positive mirroring (prizing, approval, admiration). As the mirror and idealising transferences are mobilised, the empathic, approving stance of the therapist facilitates the laying down of self-esteem regulating structures in the client.

Stolorow et al. (1987) build on the insights of Kohut; indeed, they contend that the empathic presence of the analyst is the critical factor in effective analysis. They reject the view of classical psychoanalysis in which the analyst is seen as a detached, objective observer engaged in the 'archaeological' work of excavating archaic repressed material. Instead, they construe the analytic encounter as a dialogue between two subjectivities. Rather than interpreting analysis through a reference to the intrapsychic world of the analysand on the one hand and the interpretive skill of the analyst on the other, Stolorow and his colleagues think in terms of an 'intersubjective field' set up between the two partners in the therapeutic project.

They reject the old 'rule of abstinence' (according to this rule, the analyst must refrain from providing any gratification of the patient's instinctual urges as this militates against the attempt to bring the repressed material into consciousness). In its place, they put 'sustained empathic inquiry' (Stolorow et al. 1987, p.10). Such a stance, they suggest, establishes the analyst as 'an understanding presence with whom early unmet needs can be revived and aborted developmental thrusts reinstated' (p.11).

Maurice Friedman and Richard Hycner have developed what they call a 'dialogical' approach to therapy (Friedman 1985, 1992, 1998; Hycner 1991). Like a number of adherents of the relational approach, they are inspired by Buber's teaching, particularly his understanding of 'healing through meeting'. The dialogue between therapist and patient Buber (1990) characterises this way:

> In a decisive hour, together with the patient entrusted to and trusting in him, [the psychotherapist] has left the closed room of psychological treatment in which the analyst rules by means of his systematic and methodological superiority and has stepped forth with him into the air of the world where self is exposed to self. There, in the closed room where one probed and treated the isolated psyche according to the inclination of the self-encapsulated patient, the patient was referred to ever-deeper levels of his inwardness as to his proper world; here outside, in the immediacy of one human confronting another, the encapsulation must and can be broken through, and a transformed, healed relationship must and can be opened to the person who is sick in his relations to otherness – to the world of the other which he cannot remove into his soul. (p.142)

Informed by this vision, Friedman (1998) describes 'dialogical psychotherapy' as 'a therapy that is centered on the *meeting* between the therapist and his or her client...as the central healing mode, whatever analysis, role playing, or other therapeutic techniques or activities may also enter' (p.27).

Hycner is a Gestalt therapist who declares an interest in the relationship between the intrapsychic and the interpersonal. He argues, following the Jungian therapist Hans Trüb, that intrapsychic conflict or neurosis is really a 'flight from meeting' (Hycner 1991, p.56). In dialogical work, the therapist aims to be both a real person and a 'proxy' for the world. That is, she uses the therapeutic relation to repair the dialogical bridge between the client and the community.

These therapists, then, cover a wide spectrum of psychotherapeutic theory. They indicate, moreover, that they happily use the techniques in which they were trained. What indicates their dialogical orientation is the conviction that *the therapeutic relationship is primary*. While they all recognise the benefits in using technical interventions when it seems appropriate, they are convinced that the most potent factor in promoting improvement is the capacity of the therapist to facilitate a genuine relationship with the client. In this facilitation, she brings her compassion, availability, empathy and wisdom. For the proponents of relational psychotherapy self-communication is indeed a virtue.

What I have been trying to do is to identify schools of thought in the four human service professions chosen for consideration which value self-communication. While they do not use our term, we have encountered a number of correlates. We have worked with words such as 'presence', 'empathy', 'affirmation', 'dialogue', 'attunement', 'encouragement' and 'respectfulness'. What we have seen in our analysis is that leading theorists in our four fields are contending that it is these personal qualities and attitudes which are central in achieving core professional aims. Using MacIntyre's framework, self-communication is the personal excellence which moves those involved in the personal service practice towards the goods internal to that practice. In human service, self-communication is a virtue. It is possible, then, to discern a very clear religio-ethical dimension in certain contemporary human service theories.

The natural and the Christian virtue in self-communication

I have been saying in a variety of ways that in personal service availability to the other is a virtue. In attempting to live faithful to Christ's call to 'neighbour-love', Christians will want to operate agapically in their professional life. But Christians do not, of course, have a monopoly on love and self-communication. It seems important to ask, then, whether there is a difference between natural and Christian expressions of the virtue of self-communication.

We saw in the previous chapter that Aquinas described a virtue unrelated to a supernatural end as incomplete, imperfect. Moral virtues which produce good deeds directed to a proximate, temporal end may be called true virtues, but they lack the perfection which comes from an orientation to the complete, total happiness of the beatific vision. This view raises the issue of what Bonnie Kent has called 'moral provincialism' (Kent 1994). According to this perspective, natural virtue is somehow inferior to Christian virtue.

Aquinas' distinction between imperfect and perfect virtue is grounded in his understanding of the relationship between nature and grace. For Aquinas, grace is a kind of superstructure added on to nature. Through grace, God infuses faith, hope and love into human nature, thereby transforming it and orientating it to God. Life comes in two stages. A person exists in a natural state without God. In a moment of grace, she enters a second stage, the stage that represents her movement towards the ultimate end of her existence. With this view of the relationship between nature and grace, it is inevitable that the moral life would be distinguished in terms of incomplete (natural) and complete (supernatural) virtue.

There is another view of nature and grace, however, one which I judge to be superior, namely that represented by Karl Rahner's notion of the 'supernatural existential' (Rahner 1961). Using it as a basis, we are able to transcend the moral provincialism in Aquinas. Rahner argues that there is an existential in the human (in every human) which is a 'potency', a capacity for grace, for God's self-communication in love. Grace is at the heart of our existence in freedom and knowledge. This offer can be accepted or rejected (the human is free and God has freely offered it). The supernatural existential factor determines our being ontically (with reference to the order of being) and ontologically (in terms of our concrete existence in the world). Moreover, it determines our existence *a priori*, transcendentally. That is, even when the offer is refused it continues to shape and define what it is to be human and to live in this world. It is this capacity for grace, then, that is the defining factor in human existence.

While Rahner wants to locate the human person in the supernatural order (she has this inherent receptivity for God's offer of grace), he also wants to protect the gratuity in God's offer of grace. It cannot be the case that God is robbed of God's freedom in relation to grace. God cannot be placed under a compulsion to give God's love and mercy. Now if the offer of grace is to be unexacted (not owed to the human), the existential itself must be unexacted. That is, the supernatural existential which is God's offer of grace must be something which the human can freely accept or reject.

We see, then, the contrast between this view of the relationship between nature and grace and that of Aquinas. The supernatural existential means that the human in her essential being is constituted by an offer of grace. Grace is not an alien reality, something which comes as completely new and different. This existential is a modification of the human spirit resulting in an ontological drive to God's grace and love. Even before a person self-consciously grasps hold of the gift of grace, the offer stamps and determines her nature.

Whenever a person experiences his transcendence, his limitless openness, through absolute fidelity to the dictates of conscience, through a patient and focused commitment to the demands of love and justice, through the disciplined, courageous choices demanded by the virtuous life, he experiences the offer of grace. A 'yes' to himself, a 'yes' to his transcendence, is also a 'yes' to the grace of the One who has drawn near to him. He has experienced an 'anonymous movement' towards God by grace (Rahner 1969). There are, then, both implicit and explicit responses to the offer of grace.

This idea of an 'anonymous faith' has obvious and important implications for our theological perspective on the virtue of self-communication. If natural and Christian expressions of self-communication are both movements towards grace – the one implicit, the other explicit – it is inappropriate to refer to the former as imperfect or incomplete virtue (even if it is granted that it is a true virtue). I contend that what distinguishes Christian from natural self-gifting is not the fact that it is consciously orientated to the perfect happiness of eternal life – both forms are in fact a movement towards God's grace – but the particular *vision* determining it. Vision is, in fact, an important notion in virtue ethics. Stanley Hauerwas, for example, has argued that vision is the primary determinant of the moral life: 'The moral life is fundamentally the life of vision, for the task is to see accurately the nature of the world, the self, and the other without illusion' (Hauerwas 1981, p.2). The way a Christian sees that which constitutes life and the world will have a profound impact on his moral life in general and on his way-of-being-with in particular. There are certain images, symbols and metaphors contained within the Christian vision of self-communication which give that vision its uniqueness and particularity. In a discussion of self-communication as a natural and a Christian virtue, this is where the focus should be. If we take Rahner's conception of the supernatural existential seriously, it is not possible to speak of natural self-communication cut off from God's offer of grace. It is therefore not appropriate to contrast Christian availability as an expression of perfect virtue with natural availability as representing imperfect virtue.

Given this idea of vision as the key category, what are some of the elements in the Christian way of seeing self-communication? I suggest that a Christian perspective on dialogue is characterised by (a) an explicit openness to God's loving self-communication, (b) a vision of Christ in the other, and (c) an awareness that the other is a potential partner in the beatific vision. This list, it goes without saying, is not exhaustive. However, it will perhaps serve to illustrate the idea that Christian vision distinguishes Christian from natural self-communication.

In an act of self-disposal in love, a person realises herself, actualises her being. The self that is turned in on itself is deformed. One that is orientated to others, on the other hand, experiences wholeness and actuality. From the perspective of theological existentialism, this self-realisation has a transcendent dimension. This process of coming to herself through self-disposal ultimately takes a person out of herself and projects her into the ground of her existence, God. Every act of self-offering is at the same time an experience of the divine self-communication. A committed disposal of the self is grounded in God's gift of grace and love.

A Christian is aware that all her efforts to be present to the other – those marked by courage and extension of her powers of love, as well as those which are fearful, weak and failing – are ultimately embraced by the love of God. In the waxing and waning of human powers of self-communication, the reality of God's enabling grace is not always in the forefront of consciousness. Sometimes the inadequacy of our self-gifting seems to belie the reality of God's empowerment in love. The fact that shapes the Christian vision of self-communication, however, is that in every act of human availability God communicates love, which really means that God gives Godself.

The presence of God in dialogue is given a sharp focus in the conviction that Christ is in the other. The gift of the self for the other is also a gift to Christ. 'I tell you the truth,' said Jesus, 'whatever you did for the least of these brothers and sisters of mine, you did for me' (Matt 25:40). Whether it is hugging a leper in Assisi or tending the sores of a homeless person on the streets of Calcutta, the saints of the church have been inspired by the vision of Christ in the suffering one. A loving person is able to look beyond that which screams out at him – physical degradation and even ugliness – to the hidden presence of Christ. In a less dramatic context, persons who are available are able to see something past the dullness, ignorance or annoying mannerisms of their companions. It is not the case, however, that this real person with her real needs is somehow unimportant in comparison with the Christ within her. A gift of the self to that person is not simply a means to the end of gifting our Lord. Rather, a vision of Christ within orientates us to the ineffable dignity and value in each and every person. It is this awareness which profoundly shapes (or should shape) our way of being with the other.

Finally, it is part of the Christian vision to contemplate the other as a potential partner in eternal glory.[3] It is, of course, the case that we know very little in a concrete sense about life in the eternal realm. And so, the author of the First Letter of John tells us that while we know we are the children of God, 'what we will be has not yet been made known' (3:2). However, we do know, he says, that we will be like Christ when he appears. Accordingly, Paul tells us that our earthly bodies characterised by dishonour and weakness will be transformed into eternal bodies marked by glory and power (I Cor 15:43). Transformed in our bodies, we will stand before the throne of God joining in the eternal hymn of praise (Rev 7:11–12). Worship is the natural response when in the immediate presence of the divine glory and majesty.

This is the glorious experience we will share with our companions in the beatific vision. Given our limited perspective, how exactly we will relate to one another cannot be fully known. This fact is of little consequence in the context of our present inquiry. The very fact that the person I am with now may be my companion in the eternal beatitude should significantly affect my perspective on my relationship with her. The gift of my self is a gift that might be for ever. My meagre offering of love and fidelity is set in an eternal context. It behoves me to offer myself with the kind of intensity and integrity befitting a relationship with such a glorious end in view.

In describing the personal availability which is a virtue in the human service professions, we referred to a number of terms. We saw that scholars in the various fields regularly use words such as empathy, compassion, presence, warmth, attunement, support, encouragement and affirmation in discussing relational capacity. There is one term, however, which is very rarely, if ever, included, and that is charm. Since I believe that charm is a very important element in the self-communication required of human service practitioners, it will receive a separate treatment in the next chapter.

Notes

1   The three rubrics I offer are intended to encapsulate the meaning in Bruner's rather lengthy descriptors: 'Seeing children as learning from didactic exposure: The acquisition of propositional knowledge'; 'Seeing children as thinkers: The development of intersubjective interchange'; and 'Children as knowledgeable: The management of "objective" knowledge'.

2   In my discussion of the relational orientation in psychotherapy, I do not attempt to include all possible representatives. Rather, it is sufficient, I believe, to identify a few major figures in the various schools. For more comprehensive surveys, see Friedman (1985, chs 2–9) and Hycner (1991, ch.7).

3   I am here borrowing from Josef Pieper in his insight that the Christian virtue of love operates within the perspective that the one loved is a potential companion in the glory of life eternal (see Meilaender 1984, p.31).

CHAPTER 4

Charm in Human Service

In the last chapter, we discussed the value of self-communication in the human service professions. We assigned a central role in nursing care, midwifery, education and psychotherapy to empathy, compassion, attentiveness and affirmation. Here we will also consider a communication of the self. However, it is a giving of self which is more elusive, more difficult to define. What is charm, really? Words such as 'attractive', 'delightful' and 'engaging' are commonly used to describe it. While these meanings are included in the kind of charm we will be considering, it is necessary to go deeper. Through his existential analysis, Marcel helps us do this. He refers to charm as 'all that is most metaphysical in the personality', as 'the quality which is doubtless only another facet of what we call existence' (Marcel 1952, p.301). The charm which I will be arguing is of value in human service not only engages and delights, but makes a more significant contribution to a person's life. It is *revelatory* and *revitalising*. When the other makes her presence felt, I am able to understand myself more clearly and fully. She highlights for me certain essential parts of my personality. Her contact 'reveals me to myself' (Marcel 1950, p.205). Further, her lively presence energises me for a more joyful, vital and hopeful engagement with life. I find my inner self revitalised.

It is important to identify the fount from which charm flows. Charm is, of course, associated with personal qualities and traits such as wit, style and grace. I want to suggest, however, that we need to look deeper to find its real source or sources. A person of charm, I will argue, is one who lives in and through a unity of *agape* and *eros*. *Agape* is expressed through an act of self-denial in which one's own needs and desires are temporarily suspended in order to attend to the other person. *Eros* produces a passion for life, for others, for God. It is a physical and spiritual energy that animates a person and renders her attractive and engaging.

We all want to be attractive and engaging. The danger for those of us lacking confidence is that we will try to manufacture charm. But it is not something which can be forced. It can only come when one is acting freely and spontaneously. Most of us, though, at some point lack confidence in our ability to make a positive impact. In the classroom, for example, we find ourselves striving to be 'cool' to engage more fully with our students. Or in the wards, we would like to be a little more lively and fun and so we catch ourselves acting out. Here Martin Buber's analysis of the difference between 'being' and 'seeming' is helpful. Buber suggests that it takes courage to be spontaneous and authentic with the other. The fall into seeming is fundamentally an act of cowardice. While it is no doubt true that it takes courage to 'be', to be real, I will be arguing that the really crucial issue is finding the self-acceptance which overcomes shame and self-doubt. Increasing our capacity for a free flow of charm comes with making the journey to the essential self. When we move towards our deepest self, make contact with it, accept and befriend it, then we are free to be that self with others.

I began above by observing that charm is a reality which is elusive, difficult to catch with words and concepts. Our first task is to attempt to do just that. Here we will draw upon Marcel's wisdom. We will see that he links charm very closely to making one's presence felt.

Charm and presence

Marcel offers a stimulating and insightful analysis of charm. In his discussion, he touches on four fundamental truths. First, charm cannot be forced or manufactured. Second, the nature of charm cannot be captured through a reference to particular traits or qualities. That the experience of charm is subjective is the third truth lifted up by Marcel. However, he hastens to add that this fact does not diminish its importance; charm is at the heart of the life of intersubjectivity. That this is the case is evident when one takes into account the fourth truth presented by Marcel, namely that charm is an important way in which a person makes her presence felt.

Marcel began his systematic reflection on the nature of charm in his *Metaphysical Journal* (hereafter referred to as *MJ*) and continued it in

Volume One of his *The Mystery of Being* (hereafter referred to as *MB*). In the *Journal*, he begins by observing that charm is a grace; it 'appears to decline with the decline of the gratuitous element in behaviour, or when a person's attention is more and more taken up with precise and specifiable ends' (*MJ*, p.300). If one tries to will charm, the result is a tension that militates against one's attempt to be charming. It cannot be forced or manufactured; it is 'the presence of the person round what he does and what he says' (*MJ*, p.301).

While one can readily identify certain qualities in a particular person that make her charming, it is not possible to generalise and say that wherever one finds qualities x, y and z one finds charm. In the end, charm is beyond conceptualisation; it is that elusive factor that makes for what Marcel elsewhere refers to as a 'lively' person (*MB*, p.139). The really alive person has a 'taste for life' and showers it around him; so that quite apart from any talents possessed or achievements recorded his presence is engaging and stimulating.

Of course, while one person may find herself drawn to what is for her a lively person, another will experience a blockage, a sense of alienation. There is a subjective dimension to the experience of charm. But for Marcel this does not mitigate its importance. Charm has a place at the heart of intersubjective experience:

> And the very fact that charm, which is the expression of a presence, works in some conditions and not in others, for some people and not for others, underlines the non-objective character of the notion of presence. *Non-objective* does not, however…really in the least mean *merely subjective*, in the privative interpretation of that phrase; it does not mean being more or less of the nature of an intermittent hallucination. Instead of subjectivity, we should think of intersubjectivity. Charm is non-objective but it is intersubjective. (*MB*, p.207)

Thus, for Marcel, charm cannot be considered as merely incidental to human existence. He makes the bold claim that charm can be linked 'with all that is most metaphysical in the personality, with the quality which is irreducible and incapable of being objectivised – the quality which is doubtless only another facet of what we call existence' (*MJ*, p.301).

Although Marcel does not explicitly say so, the 'metaphysical' quality of charm is associated, I suggest, with the fact that it has an important role in establishing 'communion'. When a person makes his presence felt, observes Marcel, I experience communion with him.

> We can…have a very strong feeling that somebody who is sitting in the same room as ourselves, sitting quite near us, someone whom we can look at and listen to and whom we could touch if we wanted to make a final test of his reality, is nevertheless far further away from us than some loved one who is perhaps thousands of miles away or perhaps, even, no longer among the living. We could say that the man sitting beside us was in the same room as ourselves, but that he was not really *present* there, that his *presence* did not make itself felt. But what do I mean by presence, here? It is not that we could not communicate with this man… Yet something essential is lacking. One might say that what we have with this person, who is in the room, but somehow not really present to us, is communication without communion: unreal communication, in a word. He understands what I say to him, but he does not understand *me*… By a very singular phenomenon indeed, this stranger interposes himself between me and my own reality, he makes me in some sense also a stranger to myself; I am not really myself while I am with him.
>
> The opposite phenomenon, however, can also take place. When somebody's presence really does make itself felt, it can refresh my inner being; it reveals me to myself, it makes me more fully myself than I should be if I were not exposed to its impact. (*MB*, p.205)

While Marcel says that we should not regard charm and presence as simply identical, he posits a very close link (*MB*, p.207). Charm is an important way in which a person makes his presence felt. It is 'the presence of the person round what he does and what he says'. It is the lively, stimulating way he engages with others. It is at the centre of all intersubjectivity.

We may now have some idea of what charm is and of its crucial role in interpersonal life. But there is another question, one which is equally as difficult to answer, and that is: From whence does charm spring?

Charm and the unity of *agape* and *eros*

There are certain traits and qualities which are commonly associated with charm. Most people find themselves engaged by wit, liveliness and warmth. Grace, panache and style are also qualities that many would link to charm. In order to identify the source of the power to reveal and revitalise, however, I suggest that we need to go deeper. I contend that it is when a person lives in and through a unity of *agape* and *eros* that her presence is truly stimulating, renewing and revelatory (in the sense of revealing the self of the other to herself).

In its fullest sense, *agape* refers to an impartial self-giving for the sake of the other. One spends oneself for the other not because one is attracted to him, or because he has done anything to merit it, but simply because he is someone made by God and someone Christ died for. I am interested here in a particular expression of *agape* – namely, the suppressing of one's own needs and desires in order to attend fully to the other. This, as we saw in Chapter 1, is what Marcel refers to as being hospitable, inviting the other *chez soi*. Nouwen (1972) has independently developed this notion of showing one's love for the other by affording him hospitality. An important element in a hospitable presence is a capacity for *concentration*. That is, one needs to be able to pay attention to one's guest without 'intention'. There is a giving of the self in listening and attempting to understand which is free of an intention to get something from the other. One affirms and prizes the other in and through the conversation not because one is seeking some reward, but simply because a guest deserves special treatment. I would want to add – Nouwen is no doubt completely aware of this – that none of us are capable of completely dismissing selfish intentions. We almost always look for a reward. 'Intention' will be there virtually all the time, but if it dominates our encounters with others we are not hospitable people. And nor are we very charming (in the sense I am intending). We may have style, wit and grace, but if we have little or no capacity to 'concentrate' on the other, she will not feel refreshed and renewed in her inner being. She may have been entertained, she may have laughed quite a bit, but she will not have experienced communion. In communion, something in the other touches the soul and revitalises it. This can only happen if he is a person who lives in and through *agape*.

But is *agape*-love sufficient to generate charm? It is possible to have a saintly tendency to temporarily suppress one's own needs and desires in order to attend fully to others while at the same time being quite dull and bland. If at one end of the spectrum there is the 'egocentric entertainer', at the other end there is the 'dull altruist'. In a provocative and challenging essay entitled 'Moral Saints' (hereafter referred to as *MS*), the moral philosopher Susan Wolf sets her sights on the latter type (Wolf 1982). She defines a moral saint as 'a person whose every action is as morally good as possible, a person, that is, who is as morally worthy as can be' (*MS*, p.419). There is a variety of characters compatible with the ideal of moral sainthood. They may be more or less jovial, more or less garrulous, more or less athletic. What distinguishes them from others committed less fully to the ideal of moral perfection is that they express the standard moral values at an exceedingly high level. Thus, we have the following picture of a moral saint:

> He will be patient, considerate, even-tempered, hospitable, charitable in thought as well as in deed. He will be very reluctant to make negative judgments of other people. He will be careful not to favor some people over others on the basis of properties they could not help but have' (*MS*, p.421)

Above I said that qualities such as consideration, hospitality and charity are necessary if a person is to have charm. There is no charm, I suggested, in someone who may be witty and engaging but who has little or no care or concern for others. Wolf, however, wants to say that a moral saint may be very, very good, but will also be 'unattractive' (*MS*, p.421) and live 'a life strangely barren' (*MS*, p.419). The problem according to Wolf is that the abundance of moral values the saint has are 'apt to crowd out the nonmoral virtues, as well as many interests and personal characteristics that we generally think contribute to a healthy, well-rounded, richly developed character' (*MS*, p.421). Along with doing those things which enhance the physical, emotional and spiritual well-being of others, the person with a well-rounded and rich character makes time for non-moral interests such as literature, music, art and sport. There is no doubt that a moral saint will be 'very, very nice', but, suggests Wolf, '[the] worry is that, as a result, he will have to be dull-witted, or humorless, or bland' (*MS*, p.421). We may appreciate the saintliness and goodness of, say, a Mother Teresa or a Gandhi (Wolf does not make these specific references), but we also value 'Katherine Hepburn's grace, Paul Newman's "cool"' and 'the high-spirited passionate nature of Natasha Rostov' (*MS*, p.422).

While Wolf is right to highlight the importance of a well-rounded and rich character, she goes astray when she suggests that saints often lack such a character. It is true that some of the saints – and here I am thinking of sainthood as a religious phenomenon – were overly serious and prone to melancholy, but most had a personal presence which was deeply attractive to those who knew and loved them. As Adams (1987) points out, it was not dull-wittedness or blandness which was characteristic of the lives of the saints, but rather 'an exceptional capacity for joy' (p.165). He also correctly observes that most, if not all, of them had a charisma which inspired others to leave everything and follow them. The saint who grounds her life in God is not driven by the kind of compulsive need to do good at every turn that Wolf refers to. They are free to pursue non-moral activities because they are of the conviction that ultimately good rises up in the world not through one's own willpower and effort but through the agency of limitless, ever-present Love. Saints 'commonly have time for things that do not *have* to be done, because their vision is not of needs that exceed any possible means of satisfying them, but of a divine goodness that is more than adequate to every need' (Adams 1987, p.168). Further, a saintly life is one which is shaped and guided by the concerns and interests of God. God is not only interested in moral commands; God also delights in art, literature, athleticism, music and many other things besides. It may well be that fully submitting one's life to God involves a pursuit of one or more of these activities.

I contend that far from being dull-witted, unattractive and bland, the saint is a lively person who has a passion for life, for others, for God. Not only are they filled with *agape*, they are also energised by *eros*. As Plato says in the *Symposium*, *eros* is a longing or a desire for something or someone. A basic and universal desire, according to Plato, is for the beautiful. But the beautiful and the good are one and the same: 'Then if Love needs beautiful things, and if all good things are beautiful, he will need good things too' (1997, 201c). Happiness (a rendering of the Greek word *eudaimonia*, which has no exact English equivalent) is found when one possesses good and beautiful things. The way of happiness or blessedness is a spiritual ascent which begins with a sensuous experience of the beautiful, passes through the beauty of customs and ideas, and finally reaches the heavenly realm of the Forms:

> This is what it is to go aright, or be led by another, into the mystery of Love: one goes always upwards for the sake of this Beauty, starting out from beautiful things and using them like rising stairs: from one body to two and from two to all beautiful bodies, then from beautiful bodies to

beautiful customs, and from customs to learning beautiful things, and from these lessons he arrives in the end at this lesson, which is learning of this very Beauty, so that in the end he comes to know what it is to be beautiful. (211c)

It is *eros* which supplies us with a certain physical and spiritual energy. Our desires and longings are the source of our passion for life and ultimately for God. *Eros* is 'a creative energy, the life force, the unifier, the creative urge in nature and the human spirit...' (Avis 1989, p.129). The person who has 'a taste for life' and showers it around (Marcel) opens herself to the power of *eros*. There is a joy, a radiance, an engaging physical and spiritual presence in the person living in the power of *eros*-love. Behind *eros* as a source is the passionate love of God. On this the moral philosopher Donald Evans is eloquent. God is the fount of a 'pervasive energy' in human beings which does the work of

> inspiring their most creative passions, transfiguring their faces with generous radiance, animating their movements with the graceful dance of life, uniting them with me and with all creatures, breaking down our isolation from one another, and liberating each of us to be truly ourselves. (Evans 1980, p.104)

It is this passion, grace and radiance that gives expression to charm. Persons who engage, delight and renew us not only have a capacity for setting themselves aside to attend to us, they also live in the power of desire and longing. The introduction of the idea of desire may lead some to think that *eros* ultimately refers to an inordinate self-love. Our most authentic desires, though, are not ultimately focused on self but involve a reaching out to others. This is so because they reflect God's desire that all people may know the healing, renewing, saving power of God's love.

The classic statement of rejection of any attempt to build a unity of *agape* and *eros* is provided by Anders Nygren in *Agape and Eros* (1932, 1939). For him, the two themes 'agree no better than fire and water' (Nygren 1939, p.254). According to Nygren, *agape*-love involves 'self-spending and self-offering', *eros*-love is ultimately egocentric. The Platonic vision of securing the Good through an ascent from the world of sense to the world above is one which is in the final analysis centred on the self. 'The very fact,' Nygren (1932) writes, 'that Eros is a love of desire is sufficient to show its egocentric character; for every desire of the self is a desire of good for the self' (p.137). Nygren rejects all attempts to reconcile the two loves.

Contrary to Nygren, I believe that it *is* possible to conceive of a love that incorporates both *agape* and *eros*. In attending to our deepest desires we reach not a point of self-absorption but rather the essential self. The journey inward to the real self is also a movement into God. Here I find the reflections by the Jesuit Philip Sheldrake most helpful. He suggests that 'at the heart of all of us is a centre that is a point of intersection where my deepest desire and God's desiring in me are found to coincide' (Sheldrake 1994, p.17). As I have already mentioned, God's desire is for healing, renewal and liberation for all, including the one on this journey inwards. The quest, of course, is to move beyond all the superficial, distracting desires to reach the level of authentic desire. To reach that level is not an achievement but a grace. The Spirit of Christ leads us on the journey. Importantly, as Sheldrake (1994, p.78) points out, we cannot simply leap over the many desires to reach the deepest desire. It is not as if by a massive effort of will, through sustained prayer and contemplation, one can simply sift out all the surface desires until one is left with only that desire that really matters. In real life, we engage with a variety of longings. Sometimes we find ourselves utterly confused; often we are very distracted; we wish there were a simpler, less painful way to reach the essential self. We need to learn to use the many desires as 'staging posts on a journey towards what is most true in us' (Sheldrake 1994, p.78).

I mentioned immediately above that finding the essential self, the self in the image of God, is a grace and not an achievement. In Augustine's (1991) attempt to unify *agape* and *eros* in Chapter VII of the *Confessions*, he associates a reliance on grace in reaching out for all that is good and beautiful, including the ultimate locus of good and beauty, with humility. He acknowledges the role of *eros* in leading him in the heavenly ascent from bodies to the soul, and from there to the power of reasoning (xvii [23]). In reflecting on the power of thinking he became aware that it is changeable. But the unchangeable must be superior to the changeable. 'So in the flash of a trembling glance it attained to that which is' (xvii [23]). Augustine reports that he was not strong enough to hold onto the vision of God. It was pride which kept him from God: 'My swelling conceit separated me from you, and the gross swelling on my face closed my eyes' (viii [11]). Despite their benefits to him, the Neoplatonists could not show

Augustine the way of humility. To ascend to the world of the Forms is for them an achievement, and one in which one can take great pride. The kenotic way, emulating the One who was in the form of God but who chose to take on the form of a servant and empty himself, is something they know nothing of (viii [14]). While he learned a great deal from the Neoplatonists, much of which reflects the teaching of the scriptures, he could not learn from them the truth that finding the spiritual path is a grace:

> I began reading and found that all the truth I read in the Platonists was stated here [in the scriptures] together with the commendation of your grace, so that he who sees should 'not boast as if he had not received' both what he sees and also the power to see. (xxi [27])

The key insight for Augustine is that the arrogance of knowledge separates us from God and keeps us from the path of humility and love:

> I prattled on as if I were expert, but unless I had sought your way in Christ our Saviour (Titus 1:4), I would have been not expert but expunged. I began to want to give myself airs as a wise person. I was full of my punishment, but I shed no tears of penitence. Worse still, I was puffed up with knowledge (I Cor. 8:1). Where was the charity which builds on the foundation of humility which is Christ Jesus? (xxi [26])

This is an important reflection in the context of our attempt to unite *agape* and *eros* as the twin founts of charm. Augustine is concerned with the role of humility and love in finding God. But his thoughts also have an important application in interpersonal encounters. A person filled with physical and creative energy, radiant and stimulating, may still be 'puffed up' with pride. There is a wall that separates her from all but the interesting and the intelligent. When she chooses the way of humility and charity, however, she is able to reach out to others, including the less attractive. She does not consider herself better than those she meets; rather she believes that everyone is worthy of her hospitality. All people have a fundamental dignity as persons created by God and saved by God through the loving act of Christ. In upholding that dignity, she aims to make those she encounters feel special, valuable. Her grace, humour and liveliness are not reserved simply for those who can reciprocate. Rather, she wants to use her charm to enrich and renew everyone she meets.

I hope that I have been able to demonstrate the central role of charm in intersubjectivity. Charm is not a superficial phenomenon, but something which is tied into the power of love. It is important in establishing a communion which revitalises the spirit and allows us to enter into life with renewed vigour and hope. I have yet to show, however, that charm has an important function not just in interpersonal encounters in general, but in personal service in particular.

The value of charm in human service

A nurse enters a room and just her very presence 'lights up' the room for the patients. During a day which is characterised by discomfort and dreariness her charm is greatly valued. It makes the day a little easier to bear. More than that, it brings with it joy and hope. Or, alternatively, think of the teacher who is loved by his pupils. They have come to know his characteristic phrases, gestures and routines so well. There is that warm look he gets when he is particularly pleased, the way his face lights when he is talking about matters he deems to be of great value and importance, and his good use of humour. Despite moments when they are angry with, or bored by, him, on the whole the students enjoy sharing the day with their teacher. They feel that they really belong in his classroom, that it is a good place to be. I believe that in these cases we have illustrations of what Marcel means by the capacity of charm to 'refresh [the] inner being' of a person. Through the personal contacts that are part of their jobs, some people enable others to enter into their activities, into life, with increased joy, anticipation, vitality and hope.

Marcel also refers to a 'revelatory' capacity in charm. The engaging presence of the other 'reveals me to myself, it makes me more fully myself than I should be if I were not exposed to its impact' (Marcel 1950, p.205). It is somewhat more difficult to interpret what Marcel means by this statement than by his reference to the renewing power of charm. We naturally think of an encounter with a charming person as refreshing. But what does it mean to speak of the other's presence as revealing me to myself? Marcel himself does not help us; he never elaborates on his statement. Perhaps the revelatory power in charm is connected to its capacity to 'disarm' the other. By this I mean that when we find ourselves engaged by the other, drawn into communion with him, we begin to relax our defences. We also find ourselves becoming less self-conscious. In this 'disarmed' state, we talk more freely and openly than is customary. A colleague of mine has a very warm and engaging personality. He once shared a story with me of an intimate and very significant conversation he had with a close friend. His friend was surprised at how open she was being with him: 'You're like a truth serum,' she said. 'I'm telling you things I haven't told anyone else. Why is that?' In talking freely and honestly like that we discover new and important things about ourselves. This is of course a very important factor in the psychotherapeutic relationship. There is no built-in revelatory power in therapy. The client needs to be relaxed and reassured by the presence of the therapist. That the establishing of trust and rapport in the early stages of therapy is crucially important is a commonplace in the psychotherapeutic literature. Along with compassion and empathy, I place charm as a significant factor in building rapport. The serious, largely humourless 'psycho-technician' who mechanically reflects back the client's thoughts and feelings does not encourage open and honest conversation. It is the therapist who has a 'taste for life', who is warm and personable, who is able to put her client at his ease, to lower his defences, who can do this. In the free and profound conversation that ensues, he finds his self being revealed to himself.

I do not mean to over-estimate the value of charm in human service. It is true that there are more important expressions of self-communication. In the previous chapter we discussed some of these – namely, empathy, compassion, availability and affirmation. If the value of charm should not be over-estimated, neither should it be under-estimated. Whether it is in the context of the discomfort of life in a hospital ward, or in the grind of learning, or in the pain of therapy, we need a spark of vitality and delight. We need to have our inner selves refreshed such that we might continue on the journey with renewed vigour, joy and hope.

Charm and the authentic self

Mr Jones is a dedicated and competent teacher. He considers that on the whole he relates quite well to his pupils, but he is concerned that some may think he is a little too 'stiff', a bit too old-fashioned. A decision is made to make some changes. Mr Jones attempts to project a 'more hip' image in the classroom.

Nurse Smith admires some of the other nurses who seem to be so lively and fun to be around. She is very aware of how warmly the patients relate to them. As a result, she decides to bring a little more vitality to her patient contact.

Of course, such attempts to project a desired image are futile. Charm cannot be forced or manufactured. To have it is a grace. The attempt to cultivate charm is counter-productive because it 'appears to decline with the decline of the gratuitous element in behaviour, or when a person's attention is more and more taken up with precise and specifiable ends' (MJ, p.300).

In discussing this tendency to manufacture an image, Buber (1957) refers to two fundamental human modalities, namely *being* and *seeming*. Being is grounded in 'what one really is' whereas seeming is orientated to image, impressions, appearances. The 'lie' associated with seeming, observes Buber, is not so much a distortion of facts as a falling away from spontaneity and authenticity. Buber (1957) offers a telling illustration of the confusion and deceit filling a meeting between two persons – he calls them Peter and Paul – intent on projecting an image:

> Let us list the different configurations which are involved. First, there is Peter as he wishes to appear to Paul, and Paul as he wishes to appear to Peter. Then there is Peter as he really appears to Paul – that is, Paul's image of Peter, which in general does not in the least coincide with what Peter wishes Paul to see; and similarly there is the reverse situation. Further, there is Peter as he appears to himself, and Paul as he appears to himself. Lastly, there are the bodily Peter and the bodily Paul. Two living beings and six ghostly appearances, which mingle in many ways in the conversation between the two. Where is there room for any genuine interhuman life? (p.107)

How can there be communion when all there are are 'ghostly appearances'? Buber (1957) suggests that a real meeting between two people requires courage: 'To yield to seeming is man's essential cowardice, to resist it is his essential courage' (p.108). While relating to the other as one's authentic self does require courage, the association of seeming with cowardice seems somewhat harsh. We often fail to relate to others freely and spontaneously because we lack confidence in the real self. We sense that the other will not find the self that is authentically us attractive and delightful, but rather a little boring and uninteresting. In our desperation we resort to projecting what we think will be a charming persona. The problem is not so much cowardice as shame and guilt. Henri Nouwen expresses the matter well in his discussion on the celebration of life which he describes through the metaphor of raising our cups (we make a toast to life):

> When we dare to lift our cup and let our friends know what is in it, they will be encouraged to lift their cups and share with us their own anxiously hidden secrets. The greatest healing often takes place when we no longer feel isolated by our shame and guilt and discover that others often feel what we feel and think what we think and have the fears, apprehensions, and preoccupations we have. (Nouwen 1996, p.59)

It is in coming to know, accept and befriend our real selves that we come to a point of relating freely and spontaneously with others. It is not so much a question of being courageous – although there is an element of courage associated with every genuine encounter with the other – it is more the case that when we learn to love and trust the authentic self we will be able to live out of it. An important factor in this journey to acceptance, as Nouwen observes, is overcoming the isolation which tricks us into thinking that we are the only ones who live with fear, insecurity and self-doubt. The person who has unblocked the channels through which her charm flows is the person who has journeyed to her real self and befriended it. In her personal and professional lives, she is able to shower her 'taste for life' around, enriching the lives of others all the while.

In this first part of our research, we have been concerning ourselves with various ways in which the self is communicated in human service. Our argument has been that a high capacity for self-communication is a virtue in this particular kind of work. Not only do professions such as nursing, midwifery, education and psychotherapy require high skill levels, they also demand a desire and an ability to express empathy, warmth, compassion, affirmation and charm.

We now go deeper with our analysis as we look at fundamental relational questions in the organisational life supporting the work of human service professionals. In particular, we will explore the issues of belonging and trust.

PART II

Belonging and Trust
in Organisational Life:
A Covenantal Perspective

Introduction to Part II

In this second half of the book, we will widen the scope of our concern. We will move from a consideration of the spirituality of human service acts to the moral quality of the organisational life that is the context for those acts. The aim is to see how the insights of organisational theorists concerning intelligent workplace relations apply in the particular case of human service provision.

It will be my contention that belonging and trust are critical factors in relation to the promotion of well-being in the workplace. In seeking to develop an understanding of those factors which produce a sense of belonging and which build trust, we will be hoping for 'cross-fertilisation' between organisational theory and covenant theology.

In Chapter 5, I suggest that three factors are significant in generating a sense of belonging: *recognition, responsiveness* and *identification*. In relating these factors to the covenant, I identify four theological principles which inform our understanding of belonging in the workplace. First, recognition of personhood is at least as important, and probably more important, than the recognition of achievement (Yahweh elected not a great nation but a slave people). Second, a proactive approach in attending to the needs of others heightens a sense of belonging (the covenant was founded on an initiative of grace). The third principle is that priority should be given to those most at risk (*Torah* points to a special concern for the alien, the widow and the orphan). Finally, in order to be at home in one's environment it is necessary to internalise the dominant vision (God called Israel to identify with *Torah* and now calls us to identify with the way of the Kingdom).

The theme of Chapter 6 is trust between management and staff. I suggest that *partnership* is an appropriate term for linking the realities of management–staff relations with those of the covenant relationship between Yahweh and Israel. Partnership, I will contend, is built through dialogue. Dialogue, in turn, has two fundamental requirements. First, the parties need to be able to include themselves in each other's aims, needs and aspirations. Second, they must commit themselves to working co-operatively to actualise agreements entered into. I contend that God in God's covenant activity provides an ideal for human dialogue.

In Chapter 6, we will also reflect on the nature of the highest level of trust in the workplace, namely identification-based trust. It is a form of trust in which the preferences of the other have been internalised. It will be my suggestion that in the partnership between God and Israel, and later between Christ and the church, there is a vivid demonstration of a fact which social psychologists and organisational theorists have been much more recently establishing empirically. This fact is that where there is a strong sense of group identity there is an equally strong tendency for the actors to own the corporate vision. In human service organisations (as in all other types), however, the establishment of a cohesive sense of identity is often problematic. The particular case we will look at is the clash of visions that centres on the personalist versus instrumentalist question.

In the final chapter, we will begin by considering the way in which competition, co-operation and trust function in the commercial world. The aim is to find some principles that will be useful in analysing the functioning of the British National Health Service. We will see that trust between firms can be established at two levels – namely, at the level, first, of the business system, and, second, at the level of relationships between firms. 'System power' results when a strong and effective group of trade associations, working in conjunction with the legal system, produces binding norms and standards for business. These norms and standards significantly mitigate the risk of opportunistic behaviour. In the context of the NHS, system power is established through 'clinical governance'. This system refers to the statutory duty of health care administrators to work towards optimising the level of quality in the services they provide.

Even when system power is not particularly strong, however, it is still possible to build trust. Trust is a function of the moral commitment of the various agents. In the covenant, I will be suggesting, there was both system power and personal 'investment'. Ultimately God moved the covenant from cult, *Torah* and monarchy (the elements of system power in the covenant) to a new level through an intensely personal involvement in the divine–human relationship through the incarnation and the cross-resurrection. The goal of the new life in Christ is identification with God and God's project as revealed in the Son. Covenant theology tells us, I will argue, that while system power plays an important role in establishing an environment conducive to trust, it is only through relational investment that the goal of identification with a vision is achieved.

CHAPTER 5

Belonging in the Workplace

A sense of belonging is of fundamental importance for all the agents in an organisation. In this chapter, I will be concentrating on the role it plays in the experience of human service providers. Two sources will be used in informing the discussion. The first is the general analysis of the workplace provided by organisational and other theorists. The second is covenant theology. General themes and principles drawn from these sources will be applied to the particular contexts of the personal service professions.

It is important for a staff member to feel that she is accepted and valued, that she fits in, at her place of work. When this is the case, she feels an affinity with co-workers and with the organisation as a whole. A feeling of 'at homeness' contributes significantly to a staff member's sense of well-being. Experiences of rejection, of isolation, of dissonance between personal and organisational values, by contrast, mitigate psychological welfare.

There are a number of dynamics which generate a sense of belonging in a group or community. I have singled out three central ones for attention, namely *recognition*, *responsiveness* and *identification*. 'Recognition' refers to the fact that a person feels that her value and worth has been acknowledged. 'Responsiveness' indicates the capacity in persons in positions of leadership and authority to hear and to act on the legitimate concerns of the members of the community. Finally, 'identification' captures the notion of congruence between personal and corporate values and commitments. A person is able to identify with the communal vision.

I want to explore, first, the way in which these three dynamics operated in and through the covenant established between God and God's people. The aim is to gather some theological principles which will inform and illuminate a subsequent discussion of belonging in the workplace. The four main principles are as follows. First, recognition of personhood is at least as important as, and probably more important than, recognition of achievements (Yahweh elected not a great nation but a slave people). Second, it is important not only to respond to concerns and grievances, but also to be proactive in promoting the well-being of the members of the community (the covenant was founded on an initiative of grace). The third principle is that priority should be given to those in the community who are most at risk (the concern expressed in the *Torah* for the alien, the widow and the orphan). Finally, use will be made of the notion that to be at home in one's world it is necessary to internalise a good and right vision (*Torah* and the new covenant).

Belonging in the covenant community

'I will be your God and you will be my people' is fundamentally a declaration of belonging. For the Hebrew, his or her personhood was established through the covenant. As Brueggemann (1979) puts it: '[T]he act of claiming is the act of giving life and identity to that person. Before being called and belonging to, the person was not. In the Bible, "person" means to belong with and belong to and belong for' (p.120). I suggest that the three key rubrics identified above – *recognition, responsiveness* and *identification* – capture much, if not all, of what belonging meant for the people of Israel. Let me briefly outline what I mean by these terms in the context of the covenant. 'Recognition' refers to having one's worth and value affirmed. I will be arguing that for Israel this came primarily through Yahweh's gracious election. Of all the peoples on the earth Yahweh claimed Israel as Yahweh's own. In choosing the term 'responsiveness' I have in mind Buber's (1947, pp.8–14, 45) teaching that in a relationship (in a 'dialogue') one must respond to the legitimate claims of the other (as we saw in Chapter 1, he uses the term 'responsibility'). In gracious actions God responded both to the implicit and the explicit cries from God's people. In turn, Israel was called upon to make its response to these works of grace. Finally, 'identification' refers to owning a vision or plan. We feel we belong in a community when we share its values and commitments. Israel expressed its identification with Yahweh's plan through its declaration, 'All that the Lord has said, we will do.'

Yahweh's recognition of Israel

Yahweh's loving glance, Yahweh's calling word, was responsible for Israel's existence. The originating action of Yahweh is communicated through two central narratives: the stories of the ancestors (Gen 12–36) and the Exodus–Sinai narrative (Exod 1–24). Brueggemann (1997) helpfully points out that Israel uses three verbs to express its awareness of the fact that it exists because of Yahweh's 'originary commitment': *love, choose* and *set one's heart.*

Yahweh loved the people of Israel into existence. Before God called out to them, they were no people. They had no existence, no life, no sense of belonging. To belong meant to live as the property of the Egyptian overlords. But Yahweh's love brought redemption and constituted them as a people: '[I]t was because the Lord *loved* you and kept the oath he swore to the forefathers that he brought you out with a mighty hand and redeemed you from the land of slavery, from the power of the Pharaoh king of Egypt' (Deut 7:8).

Yahweh's election of Israel is expressed most directly through the verb *choose.* The chosenness of Israel is problematic for biblical scholars and theologians. We would rather find in the Hebrew Scriptures strong indications of universal religion. Instead, we observe that Israel understood itself to be in the centre of the circle of Yahweh's salvific concern and the nations to be on the periphery. Horst Dietrich Preuss correctly points out: 'Light and shadows are both cast upon the nations, as upon Israel itself, according to the Hebrew Scriptures, and elected Israel was not finally able to come to a full expression of universal salvation' (Preuss 1996, p.303). Theologians may feel uncomfortable about this fact, but Israel certainly did not. Yahweh's act of special recognition was, on the contrary, something that it relished. In the Book of Deuteronomy we read: 'The Lord your God has *chosen* you out of all the peoples on the face of the earth to be his people, his treasured possession' (7:6b).

The verb *set one's heart* is used only twice (both times in Deuteronomy):

The Lord did not *set his affection* on you and choose you because you were more numerous than other peoples, for you were the fewest of all peoples. (7:7)

Yet the Lord *set his affection* on your forefathers and loved them, and chose you... (10:15)

The connotation in the verb is one of passionate, perhaps even sexual, pursuit (Brueggemann 1997, p.417). It is as if God were 'on the make' with Israel. Yahweh pursued Yahweh's potential partner with a love which was profoundly affirming for Israel. The people were exceedingly low in status ('the fewest of all peoples') and yet God wanted them for God's own.

Responsiveness and the covenant

The relationship between Yahweh and Israel can be construed as a dialogue. More specifically, it is a dialogue established through divine initiative and human response. Martin Buber interprets responsiveness, or 'responsibility' as he prefers, in a human-to-human dialogue as answering the other's call. He identifies a mode of human perception which he calls 'becoming aware' as the starting point in this process. Recall our discussion in Chapter 1. 'Becoming aware' is contrasted with two other perceptual modes, 'observing' and 'looking on' (Buber 1947, pp.8–10). The *observer* operates with a quasi-scientific mindset. She is interested in a careful, analytical study of the other. Her aim is to compile a comprehensive list of traits. For the purposes of observation, the other person is nothing but a bundle of characteristics. The *onlooker* is not at all interested in traits. Focusing on traits, he thinks, leads one away from one's real purpose. Looking on – the artistic perspective – involves trusting one's intuitive powers. That which is really significant about the other will show itself if only one is attentive and receptive.

Neither in observing nor in looking on, however, do we find the possibility of being addressed directly by the other. The observer perceives a bundle of traits, the onlooker an existence, but the one who is *aware* perceives a call to action, feels the weight of destiny falling on him. In 'a receptive hour', he opens himself to that call. In becoming aware of the legitimate claims the other is making, one has a moral obligation to respond with all one's being.

At the heart of the covenant is the notion that Yahweh and Israel share in a partnership, in a communion (Brueggemann 1999; Nicholson 1986; Vriezen 1970). Bound together in love, they each have their commitments and they each make their claims. There is, to be sure, an inequality in the claim-making. Yahweh is sovereign in the relationship. And yet, because the people feel that they truly belong to Yahweh, they take the liberty of crying out in complaint when they feel abandoned.

While responsiveness is clearly descriptive of Israel's involvement in the covenant, it may seem inappropriate to use the term 'response' with reference to Yahweh's action. Much of Yahweh's work on behalf of Israel is not so much response as initiative. There are occasions, to be sure, when Yahweh responds to the intercessions of the people. The covenant, however, was founded on an initiative of grace. But God's gracious initiatives, I suggest, flow from a concern to answer the deep yearnings of the people. This is clear in relation to God's promise to the Hebrew slaves of redemption and the gift of land. Naturally, they want desperately to be free, but they do not know how this could possibly come about. They do not have any inkling of who could become an agent of redemption. God takes the initiative and declares an intention to save them. In the context of an established relationship, though, the claims on Yahweh are directly put. For example, observing the experiences of surrounding nations, the people ask for a king. Further, in the time of the exile there is a protest against Yahweh's abandonment and a call for Yahweh's saving help. There are, then, four categories with which to explore responsiveness in relation to the covenant: *land, exodus, monarchy* and *exile*. As we explore these themes, we will follow the narratives as they are presented. It is recognised that the question of the historicity of the Hebrew Scriptures is a vexed one. There is considerable debate over the extent to which what we have is an ideological construct rather than an historical account. This need not concern us here. It is the theological principles associated with the narratives that we are primarily interested in.

Turning to the first theme, the promise of land has an extended history in the life of Israel. It was a gift a long time in the offering, so to speak. Even before Israel was fully constituted as a people, the promise was made. God said to Abraham and Sarah:

> Leave your country, your people and your father's household and go to the land I will show you. I will make you into a great nation and I will bless you; I will make your name great, and you will be a blessing... (Gen 12:1–2)

During the period of slavery in Egypt the need for the fulfilment of the promise becomes particularly pressing. The Hebrews find themselves suffering in a land of bondage and oppression. They cry out in anguish but it seems as if there is no one to hear their cries. There is no power of salvation on the horizon. But Yahweh is full of grace and mercy and Yahweh hears:

> I have indeed seen the misery of my people in Egypt. I have heard them crying out because of their slave drivers, and I am concerned about their suffering. So I have come down to rescue them from the hand of the Egyptians and to bring them up out of that land into a good and spacious land, a land flowing with milk and honey... (Exod 3:7–8)

The covenant is established through this initiative of grace in which Yahweh rescues the people and gifts them with a homeland. But the gift is not unconditional. If the people fail to keep the covenant, they will lose it. Israel's 'history' in Joshua–Judges–Samuel–Kings is a chronicle of infidelity and waywardness. The ensuing judgement of Yahweh brings the ultimate disaster, namely the loss of the land. Israel becomes a people scattered. It loses the foundation on which its identity was built.

The call to repentance goes out from the mouths of the prophets and Israel hears it. But repentance is not the only reaction of the people. They are not silent in their grief and desperation. Reaching into the ancient practice of lament and complaint they shout out to God. Indeed, the crying out spills over from lament into protest. The people protest against Yahweh's abandonment: 'Why have you rejected us forever, O God? Why does your anger smoulder against the sheep of your pasture?' (Ps 74:1). The fact that the people feel free to complain, to remind God of God's pledges of fidelity, indicates the strength of their sense of belonging. Israel seeks in and through its pleading to move God to saving action:

> Remember the people you purchased of old, the tribe you redeemed as your inheritance – Mount Zion, where you dwelt.

> Pick your way through these everlasting ruins, all this destruction the enemy has brought on the sanctuary.

> Your foes roared in the place where you met with us; they set up their standards as signs...

> Do not hand over the life of your dove to wild beasts; do not forget the lives of your afflicted people forever.

> Have regard for your covenant, because haunts of violence fill the dark places of the land.

Do not let the oppressed retreat in disgrace; may the poor and needy praise your name. (Ps 74:2–4, 19–21)

The expressions of grief and of protest are calling Yahweh to move beyond sovereign anger and outrage to rescue and restoration. In grace and mercy, Yahweh hears and changes the direction in the relationship from judgement to redemption. In a suggestive phrase, Brueggemann (1997) calls this 'Yahweh's inexplicable turn toward Israel' (p.441). Israel rejoices in its salvation but it does not know what has produced this change of heart.

Time and time again Israel experienced the blessing of Yahweh. The people were called upon to respond to God's grace through love and through moral and spiritual fidelity. In his excellent study of community in the Bible, Hanson (1986, p.30) observes that the 'twin human responses' were worship and *Torah*. In living faithful to *Torah*, the people manifest righteousness and compassion. 'For a community to have a heart, justice had to be infused with compassion' (Hanson 1986, pp.72–73).

In relation to belonging, both these elements are of great significance. Israel entered into communion with Yahweh in special places, in places of great beauty. The tabernacle (Exod 25:3–7) and the temple (Ps 48:2; Ps 29:2; 1 Chr 18:29; 2 Chr 20:21) traditions both highlight Israel's understanding that the beauty of God's presence calls for a beautiful place in which to host that presence (Brueggemann 1997). In these places of physical loveliness the people glorified Yahweh and celebrated their bond of love with Yahweh.

Second, Israel was a community established for the sake of justice and compassion. The Israelites were bound together in a communion in which each member was treated well enough to maintain full membership. Special consideration was required in relation to the weak and the poor:

For the Lord your God is God of gods and Lord of lords, the great God, mighty and awesome, who shows no partiality and accepts no bribes. He defends the cause of the fatherless and the widow, and loves the alien, giving him food and clothing. (Deut 10:17–18)

This demand for justice is to be seen as a foundational element in the building of a community in which the common good is advanced and all members, including the weak and the poor, have a genuine sense of belonging.

Above it was stated that in the experience of the exile we have an example of the people making a direct claim on Yahweh. In the request for a king we find another such example. There is in this call for the establishment of a monarchy a strong tension, a deep sense of ambivalence. It seemed to some that the communion with Yahweh as King would be endangered by the presence of an earthly king (1 Sam 8:7). This objection was largely overcome, however, through royal David's mighty and impressive deeds. (A convenient summary of David's achievements, which I use here, may be found in Bright 1979.) In a few short years, David transformed Israel into the dominant power in all of Palestine and Syria. The occupation of the land had been far from complete. But under David's strong leadership, control of Palestine became total. He went on to win a considerable foreign empire (encompassing the Transjordanian states of Moab, Edom and Ammon, and the Aramaean states of southern and central Syria). Though the people benefited considerably from Israel's enhanced status and prosperity, David was far from perfect. His reign reflected the less noble traits of the other ancient near-eastern monarchs. This was a monarchy that could be oppressive and self-indulgent (though the official theology tends to mask this) (Brueggemann 1999, pp.26–27).

In sum, the covenant relationship was built on a dynamic of divine initiative and human response. It may not be clear, then, that it is appropriate to refer to Yahweh's 'responsiveness'. I have suggested, though, that in taking the gracious initiative God was meeting the most pressing needs of the people. They needed liberation and they cried out in their suffering. Though it seemed to them that their utterances of pain, their desperate pleas, were simply lost in the air, God was there and God heard. There were also occasions after the covenant partnership had been established (during the exile, in the request for a king) when the pleas were explicit. Israel now knew Yahweh and felt it really belonged to Yahweh. The people took the liberty of pleading with, and even protesting to, their God. God in God's goodness and love responded in powerful ways. In the face of this abundant grace, Israel was called to respond in faith and in love. That response took the twin forms of worship and *Torah* observance. This latter form is especially important in the context of the final category for discussion, namely Israel's identification with Yahweh's will and purpose.

Belonging and identification with Yahweh's plan

As we have seen, the covenant was founded on an initiative of grace. In calling the people into relationship, Yahweh began by pointing to Yahweh's saving acts on their behalf (Exod 19:4). And the people responded by declaring their commitment: 'All that the Lord has said, we will do' (Exod 19:8). In committing itself to *Torah*, Israel indicated its identification with Yahweh's will and purpose.

Torah is usually rendered in English as 'law'. But as is routinely pointed out by scholars of the Hebrew Scriptures, this is somewhat misleading. It gives the impression that *Torah* has merely to do with formal regulations. In fact, *Torah* means pointing the way. Israel understands it as '*guidance*, in order to be joyously "on the way"...' (Brueggemann 1999, p.38).

But we know, of course, that Israel often lost its way. One possibility when it comes to countering a tendency to waywardness is the telling of stories of faithfulness. This is something the theologians who constructed the Hebrew Scriptures had very firmly in mind. They used the ancient narratives available to them in the attempt to get Israel going in the right direction again. The Deuteronomistic theologians (7th century BC), for example, looked back to the faithful actions of the ancestors when the people were under siege (Preuss 1996, p.16). In their writings, the fathers and mothers in the faith are not seen as set in a distant moment of history, but rather as part of present experience. The present community shares in the experiences of the earlier generations. These include guilt (Deut 5:9; 1 Kgs 9:9, 14:22; 2 Kgs 17:14ff; Jer 3:25, 23:27); the saving work of the exodus (Josh 24:17; Judg 2:1, 6:13; 1 Sam 12:6, 8); the gift of land (1 Kgs 14:15; 2 Kgs 21:8); and the gift of the temple (Jer 7:14). The 'God of the ancestors' is a frequent reference in these writings. It is this God who has been abandoned. Presenting the stories anew serves both to warn the people and to inspire them to a renewal of faith and practice.

The waywardness and rebelliousness of the people indicates a failure to internalise Yahweh's plan. It is this failure which prompts Yahweh to inaugurate a new covenant. The prophet Jeremiah brings the new message concerning the covenant: 'I will put my law in their minds and write it on their hearts' (31:33). Here we have 'a description of the complete internalization of the divine will that makes unnecessary the entire machinery of external enforcement' (Mendenhall and Herion 1992, p.1192). It would be incorrect, though, to suggest that there is no hint of internality in the old covenant (McComiskey 1985, p.85). Indeed, we find in the first covenant the ideal of internalising the divine instructions: 'These commandments that I give you today are to be upon your hearts' (Deut 6:6). The tension in the way the covenant is understood by Israel is not so much between externalisation and internalisation as between conditionality and unconditionality. In these different but complementary interpretations we have one which stresses Yahweh's eternal promises and one which highlights the possibility of divine curse (Bright 1979, p.25). The former was grounded in the Abrahamic covenant described in Chapter 15 of the book of Genesis. There the covenant is presented as a promissory oath on the part of God. There are no particular conditions attached to the divine promises of posterity and of greatness as a nation. It is the case, though, that it is assumed that Abraham would continue to trust, to walk with, Yahweh. Thus, it can be said that the patriarchal covenant is grounded in God's unconditional promises for the future and asks of the recipient only that he trust. The covenant at Sinai, on the other hand, had a quite different character. It was not a promissory covenant. Rather, it created a partnership between God and the people which was grounded in the gracious, saving actions God had already performed and which required obedience in order to assure the continuation of divine blessings.

It is not easy to fully reconcile these two different understandings of the covenant relationship. There is no consensus amongst biblical scholars as to how such a reconciliation might be achieved. The approach offered by Clements (1978, pp.102–103), however, is certainly plausible. Its appeal is that it offers a cogent interpretation of the reactions of the Deuteronomists to the very difficult and changing circumstances in the 7th and early 6th centuries BC. Clements begins by asking why it was that the Deuteronomic school found the blessing and curse theology of the Mosaic covenant so appealing. The only answer, he suggests, is that they saw themselves and their people as living in a period of crisis. The loss of the Northern Kingdom to the Assyrians in 722 BC, followed by the humiliation and agony of the deportations, left the great empire of David in tatters. The unthinkable was looming as a very real possibility: Israel could be annihilated completely. Hope for the future, the Deuteronomists believed, was tied to Israel learning the lessons of the past and acknowledging the extent of the threat in the present. The conditions of the salvation were consequently very fully set out. In this way, it was hoped that the people would mend their ways and step back onto the path leading to salvation.

Even as the crisis deepened and Judah's worst moment came with the fall of its king and the destruction of the temple in 587 BC, a message of hope remained for the people. Right at the centre of this message was the preaching of Jeremiah, who had projected a future for the nation (Jer 32:1–15):

> As the Deuteronomic school came to develop its covenant theology in the light of events, and with a deep consciousness of the importance of Jeremiah's preaching, so they came to look beyond the uncertainties of a conditional covenant agreement with God to the greater certainties of the divine grace and love. (Clements 1978, p.102)

There was always within the covenant an ideal of internalisation. What is novel in the new covenant is the height to which the role of divine grace is elevated. In God's love and grace, God will miraculously act to condition the minds and hearts of the people in order that they might live faithfully.

Let me attempt to summarise the discussion thus far. We have related Israel's sense of belonging in and through the covenant to three central actions on Yahweh's part. First, Yahweh *recognised* Israel through a gracious election as Yahweh's chosen ones. Second, in the course of their covenant relationship, Yahweh consistently *responded* in love to Israel's cries for help. Further, to go back a few steps, the covenant was founded on Yahweh's initiative of grace. Even before the people knew the name of their God, Yahweh reached out to meet them at their greatest points of need. Finally, Yahweh set out before Israel the vision that would shape its worship and its communal life. When they successfully *internalised* Yahweh's *Torah*, the people of Israel felt orientated in the universe. They felt at home with their God and, as a consequence, at home in their world.

In what follows, an attempt will be made to connect a sense of belonging in one's place of work with these same three rubrics: *recognition*, *responsiveness* and *internalisation*. The aim is to use covenant theology to inform and shape our understanding of what it means to feel at home in the workplace.

Belonging in the workplace

There is a range of issues which are important in relation to the sense of belonging which employees feel, or do not feel. Some researchers have, for example, pursued the question of the role of *friendship* in producing a sense of well-being in the workplace (Winstead *et al.* 1995). Others have identified both *joint projects* and *logos* as factors in creating a sense of belonging (Shapiro, Sheppard and Cheraskin 1992). Still others have theorised about the existence of an 'attraction–selection–attrition' cycle which has the effect of maintaining the climate or culture of an organisation (Schneider 1987). According to this theory, a particular organisational culture is sustained because people who identify with it are attracted to it (if they find after a time that they do not fit after all, they will leave and there is thus no chance of the culture being modified). Clearly, all these issues are important in developing an understanding of what helps people feel they belong in the place where they work. In choosing to concentrate on recognition, responsiveness and identification, I have two things in mind. First, while these are not the only issues involved, they are absolutely central. And second, it is in these areas that covenant theology makes a direct and strong contribution.

Work and recognition

We are interested here in the ways in which work functions as a validation of a person's worth and value. Fukuyama (1992) may have gone too far in his assertion that the desire for recognition is the engine which drives social, political and economic history, but he is surely right to state that the need to feel affirmed and valued as a person is highly significant in motivating people to work. There are two basic sites at which the desire for recognition *vis-à-vis* work operates. First, there is the society at large. People tend to feel that they belong in the society because they are gainfully employed. Second, there is the particular workplace or organisation. An employee feels that she belongs within an organisation when there is an appropriate recognition of her skills and of her contribution to productivity. There is another factor, however. In order to feel as though she really belongs, she must receive *personal* recognition. That is, not only must her talents and contributions be acknowledged, she must also receive validation as a person. We begin our discussion with the role of social recognition.

WORK AND SOCIAL RECOGNITION

It is widely accepted that employment is a major, and perhaps *the* major, source of belonging in the society. In relation to Israel, we saw that social citizenship was established through the claim of Yahweh (election) and participation in the ritual and social life of the nation. Today, a sense of belonging in the society is established primarily through participation in the paid workforce.

There are those, though, who want to see a change in this situation: '[D]oes the economic bond alone,' writes the philosopher Dominique Méda (1996, p.639), 'suffice to create a true sense of belonging, of belonging together, a true solidarity among the members of society?' This is an important challenge, especially given our reflections above on belonging and the covenant. In the building of its communal life, justice, compassion and a concern for the common good were key foundation stones for Israel. Méda has a vision for the building up of the contemporary society which connects quite closely with the one which Yahweh gave to the people. She launches an attack on the tendency in the sphere of economics to interpret social life in a narrow fashion. Social riches cannot be reduced to an exchange relationship which has ever-increasing levels of productivity as its sole goal.

> For economics…no value can be placed either on the existence of healthy, peace-loving, happy, civically aware, tolerant, non-violent individuals, or on the establishment of a 'good society', that is, a just, peace-seeking, closely knit and cultivated society. (Méda 1996, pp.639–640)

Méda aligns herself with that stream of philosophical thought from Hegel to Habermas which contends that social bonds are forged not only through co-operative activity in the workplace but also through collective action aimed at shaping good political institutions. Thus, for her, a high priority should be assigned by members of the society to achieving a reduction of the time taken up with work in order to allow for a fuller participation in the political process. A vigorous engagement in the political sphere offers 'the best prospect for cementing the social bond' (Méda 1996, p.641).

There is, I believe, much to recommend Méda's project. It accords with the biblical view that the primary aims in 'the good society' are not wealth creation and opportunities for material enjoyment, but rather solidarity, a mutuality in care, and the pursuit of peace and justice. Sadly, however, it seems unlikely that the vision will catch on. The challenge is just too big. Méda's idea needs an extensive and very effective educational programme if it is to begin to have an impact. Right across the board, from politicians to employers to workers, people will have to be helped to see that participation in the building of the good society should be given a much higher priority. And beyond that, workers will have to be convinced that there are viable alternatives to vocational achievements for maintaining social status. Moreover, as Méda herself acknowledges, even if people were to opt for a reduction in working hours, they would most likely devote their spare time to leisure rather than to politics. To re-orientate their thinking to incorporate a new set of values would clearly be an extremely difficult, if not impossible, task. It seems likely that for some time to come, at least, most people will continue looking to the work environment as the major source of recognition.

The social scientist Robert Castel provides an interesting and informative description of how, historically, work was assigned such a crucial role in establishing social citizenship (Castel 1996). It was at the end of the 17th century and the beginning of the 18th that the modern concept of work began to emerge. But while the economic is the major factor in our modern understanding of work, this was not the case at that time. Moral and religious considerations were also very important. Work was thought of as a path to both moral improvement and spiritual redemption.

Labour was not, however, something that was required of all persons. Those enjoying the privileges of high society also enjoyed a life of leisure. In the medieval social division, there were three estates: the clerics, the warriors and the labourers. It was only the members of the last named division who worked in the strict sense of the term – that is, laboured in the service of others. The third order originally consisted of agricultural labourers, but it was later broadened to include other occupations, along with the trades and professions. So within this broad category of the 'third estate' were, on the one side, those in the trades who were endowed with both duties and privileges and, on the other side, the unskilled workers who were seen simply as providers of a necessary, but very basic, service. While the former group were accorded due social recognition, those in the latter sector were assigned an exceedingly low status (the Frenchman Abbé

Sieyès, for example, used the term 'two-legged tools' to describe them [Castel 1996, p.617]).

Thus, observes Castel (1996, p.618), it is necessary to draw a distinction between social recognition and economic utility. In the earliest industrial enterprises, the workers provided a useful service in the project of generating new riches, but they were without social dignity. In this century, however, the activities of the labour movement, and the associated emergence of labour law, has resulted in social citizenship for the worker. She is no longer an individual at the mercy of a purely contractual order. She has the protection of both the law and of collectively engineered agreements. At the same time, of course, the workplace continues to contain within it the potential for alienation, heteronomy and exploitation. There is an ongoing struggle to ensure that the rights and the dignity of the worker are respected. This struggle is not just orientated to wage levels, important as they are. For the modern worker, issues such as balancing work and family responsibilities, workplace health and safety, control of one's work, environmental protection, gender equality and flexible working hours are also of great importance. While there have been very significant advances made, there is clearly quite a way to go in the task of fully establishing the social citizenship of the worker.

One of the reasons that people are attracted to the professions is that they guarantee a high status social citizenship. The professions offer superior rates of pay, good working conditions and high social status. In a word, the worth of a professional person is recognised by the society. With the exception of counsellors and psychotherapists, those in the human service professions we are attending to tend to feel that this is not their situation. A statement from the United Nations Fourth World Conference on Women, held in Beijing in 1995, refers to nursing as a 'low paid, low status profession' (cited in O'Connor 2002). This is difficult to dispute. The push to make nursing an all-graduate profession is one prominent reaction to this problem. Midwives are not accorded nearly the same esteem as the medical professionals they work with. Midwifery leaders are calling for a 'parity of esteem' with those professionals (O'Connor 2002). Wagner (1998) argues that the comparison should be between midwives and general practitioners, not between midwives and nurses. A lack of societal recognition is also a problem for the teaching profession. There is a widespread view that schools are under-performing and that teachers are 'out of touch' with society (Dinham and Scott 1996).

Clearly, this lack of societal recognition is a major concern. Those who represent these health and teaching professionals, together with the professionals themselves, are engaged in a long-term struggle to educate the society as to the real value of the service that is provided. In the face of a general lack of affirmation from the wider community, the importance of validation within the organisations where these professionals work is heightened.

RECOGNITION WITHIN THE ORGANISATION

It is evident that many workers place a high value on generous remuneration and offers of promotion. It may seem that here we have the primary sources of motivation for most employees. I believe, however, that Fukuyama (1992, pp.172–173, 223–234) is right when he suggests that there is a very significant 'thymotic' component in the push for higher wages and more senior posts. *Thymos* is Plato's term for the desire for recognition. It is 'something like an innate human sense of justice: people believe that they have a certain worth, and when other people act as though they are worthless – when they do not *recognize* their worth at its correct value – then they become angry' (Fukuyama 1992, p.165; emphasis in the original). A person works hard, seeks wage increases and looks for opportunities for advancement not just because he wants to be able to pay the mortgage and enjoy 'the good life'. What drives him primarily is the need to be validated as a person of worth. When a worker is not recognised through appropriate rewards he feels alienated from management and the organisation.

The thymotic dimension in work extends beyond pounds and posts, however. An employee wants not only to have her talents, initiative and productivity acknowledged; she desires also a validation of her personhood. Employees place a claim on employers to affirm their dignity and worth simply as fellow human beings. There is here a parallel with the relationship between Yahweh and Israel. Recall that what the people treasured most was the fact that Yahweh chose them not because of their collective achievements – they were a small clan living in bondage – but simply because Yahweh loved them. In the case of contemporary employment, even if the skills and achievements of workers are modest, they expect to be accorded respect and dignity. In their empirical research on the relationship between social relations at work and health, Eakin and MacEachen (1998) discuss the importance workers assign to a personalised social environment. The employees they interviewed referred to wanting to be 'treated as a person' and to the importance of employers recognising that 'employees are human too' (p.901). This concern with the personal was also communicated through the use of the family image. One worker the researchers interviewed made this comment: 'They [the owners] really look after me. Everybody's just one big happy family. It's a small company but a big happy family there...' (p.901). The language of the family was also used to communicate a valuing of acts of care and concern and of attempts to treat persons as individuals. For instance, the celebration of birthdays and other significant life events was seen to establish a family-like environment. These workers manifestly had a sense that they were considered not just as objects in a cycle of production, but as persons belonging to a 'family'.

It is important to recognise, however, that psychological well-being and a sense of belonging are not related only to the general social environment. That is, there are both individual and common components in the social climate of an organisation (Repetti 1987; Repetti and Cosmos 1991). Obviously, the general social environment impacts on the local one. But certain persons have the personality traits and social skills which elicit a relatively high number of positive responses from co-workers. So, even if the general social climate is relatively poor, some persons in the organisation will generate a positive local environment. Conversely, it may be that the overall social atmosphere is very good – it feels like 'one big happy family' – and yet a particular individual may feel as though she does not belong. Perhaps she even has a high level of job-related skill and makes a strong contribution to the organisation's output. While she appreciates the recognition she receives for her achievements, she also has a strong desire to be accepted into the workplace community. That is, not only does she want to be affirmed in her capabilities, she also wants her personhood validated.

There are, then, those persons in an organisation who lack confidence in their personal traits and qualities. It is also the case that some persons are unsure in relation to their professional skills. Or it may be that there is a lack of confidence in both areas. When there are areas in a staff member's personal and/or professional make-up which he feels are unsatisfactory, there is a temptation for him to project an image to co-workers. Perhaps he wants to be seen as more outgoing, or more sophisticated, or more efficient or more creative than he actually is. In his distorted thinking, it seems to him that to have an image recognised is better than receiving no recognition at all. He desperately wants to be accepted as a valuable member of the team, and so he resorts to projection of a persona. Afraid of 'being' he falls into 'seeming', to use Buberian language.

The strategy, of course, always fails in the end. Even if a person is successful for a time, his co-workers will eventually come to distinguish reality from appearance. That we continue to work with cover stories despite the inevitability of exposure is evidence of how desperately we seek recognition and acceptance. But as Buber (1957) suggests, the only genuine option for individuals is to come to the point where 'the will is stirred and strengthened to be confirmed in their being as what they really are and nothing else' (p.108).

The responsiveness of management

In discussing Yahweh's covenant relationship with Israel, we noted Yahweh's constant willingness to act on behalf of the people for their security, well-being and prosperity. The people of Israel felt that they really belonged with Yahweh because Yahweh demonstrated a commitment to hear and to act on their cries for salvation. There is a similar dynamic at work in contemporary workplaces. Persons feel that they belong in an organisation when those with power and authority show a genuine concern for their well-being. When management takes the legitimate claims of the staff seriously and acts accordingly, they feel an affinity with their organisation.

In what follows, three areas in which employees are seeking a positive response from management will be discussed. These are: control of one's work, achieving a balance between work and family life, and finding self-expression through one's work. Obviously there are a number of other important claims being pressed by workers today. These three issues, however, are central, and in covering them I hope to illustrate the link between managerial responsiveness and a sense of belonging.

RESPONDING TO THE CALL FOR GREATER CONTROL AT WORK

Control in the workplace has two basic dimensions: control over one's own work and control over others (Ross 1992). The latter form of control, job authority, carries with it, at least for some individuals, a degree of satisfaction. To be able to make decisions and to direct the activities of others is attractive to certain persons. For most, however, the disadvantages outweigh the advantages. The potential for frustration associated with having to rely on the co-operation of others, coupled with the possibility of conflict, renders this form of control undesirable for most. Further, the majority of employees do not have this option available to them. For these reasons, our discussion will be orientated to control over one's own work.

Occupational self-direction involves two factors. First, there is autonomy in relation to the processes associated with one's work. And second, there is the opportunity for some level of self-expression through one's work. Clearly, if a person is forced to carry out tasks in ways that she is dissatisfied with and at the same time is not given any opportunity to reshape her activities, her level of well-being will fall. Further, if the tasks she is assigned carry little or no scope for thought and independent judgement, her level of fulfilment will be very low. An employee needs an opportunity for input into the way her job is structured. Even if the scope for self-expression is relatively low, the employee herself is in the best position to determine how it can be maximised.

When an employee has little or no control over her work she feels alienated from it. Further, a lack of autonomy mitigates psychological and physical health (Andolsen 1988). If work satisfaction is low and there are negative health implications a person will feel estranged from the management and from her organisation.

Autonomous functioning is a defining feature of professional work. It is therefore interesting to note that control over one's work is often a matter of concern in the human service professions. As in the case of societal recognition, the clear exception is psychotherapy. Many therapists work in their own practices. The freedom they experience as a result is a major source of job satisfaction.

The literature on the level of control that a teacher experiences identifies two (conflicting) realities (Mander 1997). First, a teacher does in fact have a reasonable level of personal autonomy. She has a good deal of scope for developing her own particular style of teaching. A teacher must, however, contend with externally imposed directives. This clearly has the potential for significant frustration as the external directives may clash with the teacher's own preferences and commitments. This situation of dissonance may lead to a feeling of identity loss (van den Berg 2002).

Nurses work in an environment of minimal personal autonomy. Their practices are shaped to a very high degree by hospital protocols and doctor directives. Bradshaw (1999) points to a worrying trend that is associated with this feature. An unfortunate consequence of the move to make the nurse into an autonomous, academically credentialled professional may be a loss of commitment to the ethic of self-giving service. She argues that, in the trend to empowerment and assertiveness, the 'moral imperative of agape' must be maintained as the foundational principle of nursing. This view, we note, is aligned with our philosophy of nursing as self-communication.

Procedures and protocols are also a limiting factor in relation to midwife autonomy (McKay 1998). While these guidelines are often important in ensuring safety, they 'also restrict decision-making and limit innovation and flexibility' (McKay 1998, p.18). Some are of the view that autonomy is the central issue facing midwifery today (Wagner 1998). They contend that until midwives are able to work free of doctors' control, they will never be able to express their vocation fully. Indeed, it is this desire to give full expression to midwifery-led care that prompts some to establish an independent practice.

In order for a professional person to feel at home in her work environment, it is essential that she has significant scope to shape her practice around her own preferences, commitments and personal judgements. The freedom that she has can never be total, of course. There are others who have input into her professional functioning, and this is entirely appropriate. The debate is over the balance between external and internal control. Especially in the case of nursing and midwifery, there seems to be good justification for the view that external control is oppressive. In a word, these health care professionals are engaged in an emancipatory struggle.

The theological ethicist Barbara Hilkert Andolsen rightly points out the importance of addressing the problem of lack of control at work from a relational or social perspective (Andolsen 1988). Working with an individualistic framework will lead us to put the onus on the worker herself. We will tend to adopt the view that she needs to address the problem herself. For example, she could be encouraged to change her mental attitude and operate as creatively and positively as she can in the face of external control. While this may be helpful in the short term, it is not the answer.

If a relational perspective is adopted, however, the issue looks very different. For one thing, Andolsen (1988) observes, we will see the question of moral accountability in a different light. Not only is management responsible for working with nurses and midwives towards a higher level of control at work, but peak health care bodies need also to make a contribution. The struggle is painful and frustrating because these leaders, along with their political masters, currently take a different view of the situation.

In a different context, we note that Yahweh at certain points in the covenant relationship with Israel felt no obligation to respond to the plight of the people. This was because Israel had been unfaithful and had thereby given up its claim on divine grace. The time of the exile was one of desperate need for the people of God. All they could do was to cling to a faint glimmer of hope because Yahweh did not seem inclined to hear. As Brueggemann (1997) puts it: '...*Israel hoped beyond the hope or intention even of Yahweh, who had no such hope or intention for Israel*' (p.439; his emphasis). A striking feature of Israel's response to the situation, as we saw above, was its insistent pleading and protesting. Through its laments, Israel staked its claim on Yahweh in a bold and determined fashion. And eventually Yahweh heard the pleas and decided to deliver the people out of their captivity.

There is, I suggest, a strong message here for nurses and midwives. It is their commitment to collective action and their determination that their concerns must be heard by all those in positions of responsibility that are the critical factors in securing advances. Administrators, health care leaders and politicians may not feel inclined to hear, but the intensity and longevity of the protests will be difficult to resist.

RESPONDING TO THE CALL FOR A WORK AND FAMILY BALANCE

Contemporary commentators on changing patterns in the nature of employment routinely observe that a central concern for workers is achieving an appropriate balance between work and family commitments

(Herman and Gioia 1998; Mückenberger 1996; Tolbert and Moen 1998).
Employees are commonly acutely aware of their family responsibilities and
the extent to which work commitments militate against the fulfilment of
those responsibilities. Many workers are not only responsible for the care
of children and the maintenance of a relationship with a partner, they also
have commitments in the care of elderly relatives. Organisations that value
their employees and their contributions are sensitive and responsive to
these needs.

Endeavouring to keep up work and family commitments can be very
stressful. There is ample evidence that female workers are most at risk in
relation to these stressors, for they often carry the burden of a 'double day'.
The story behind women taking on an extra daily load is by now well
known to most. The pattern of the 'double day' began with the onset of
industrialisation. At that time there was a shift in the locus of certain forms
of production from the family farm to the factory or the office. To begin
with, this shift affected only relatively small numbers of women. Many,
especially those in the middle class, remained in the home, where they
continued to perform domestic and child-rearing duties. However,
throughout the 20th century there was a steady increase in the number of
women entering the workforce. Indeed, in the post-World War II era the
rise was dramatic. The fact that middle class families experienced
increasing financial expectations and/or pressures, coupled with the fact
that there were increasing numbers of clerical and service jobs available,
accounted for this flood of female workers into the labour force. A third
factor, more significant in the United States than in Britain, was the
motivation provided by the feminist ideal of economic independence. If
men had responded in large numbers to the changed situation of their
partners by increasing their involvement in domestic chores and in child
care, we would not have the phenomenon of the 'double load'. But, sadly,
any number of social surveys indicate that only a minority of males
contribute significantly in households where both adults are engaged in
paid employment. As a consequence, many women who work find
themselves having to deal with high levels of stress. They constitute an
at-risk group in the workforce.

In the covenantal ordering of communal life there was a special
concern for those most at risk, namely the alien, the widow and the orphan
(Exod 22:21–24; Deut 10:18–19; Ps 146:9; Isa 1:17). Yahweh's intention

was that all persons, especially those in a vulnerable position, receive the help and support needed to ensure their dignity and their full membership in the community. If parents, and especially mothers, are to feel fully at home in their corporate communities, they need to receive the consideration and practical assistance that will enable them to strike a sensible balance between work and family.

RESPONDING TO THE CALL FOR SELF-EXPRESSION THROUGH WORK

Writers involved in a modern interpretation of work commonly refer to the fact that a significant number of workers today are seeking after meaning in what they do (Caudron 1997; Herman and Gioia 1998). Employees increasingly are not content simply to 'attend' their workplace; they want it to be a place where they find opportunities for self-actualisation and a sense of fulfilment. Too often managers leave it too late to respond to the signs of disgruntlement and disillusionment in an employee. She may be on the verge of deciding to seek work elsewhere before any action is taken to address the problem. There is a need for management to take a proactive stance when it comes to helping workers express themselves in the workplace.

In our study of Yahweh's responsiveness in the covenant relationship, we observed that Yahweh did not always wait for a cry from the people before acting. Indeed, the covenant was founded on God's initiative of grace. Even before Israel was properly constituted as a nation, the promises of posterity and land were made to Abraham and Sarah (Gen 12:1–3). Even before the people knew the name of their God, Yahweh was compassionately studying their plight in Egypt and deciding to bring salvation.

Forward-thinking organisations are operating proactively to ensure that their employees are motivated, fulfilled and contributing optimally towards organisational aims. Leaders in these organisations see their role as going beyond being supportive of staff members in their planning for personal and professional development. They recognise that they need to take the initiative on occasion. One leader imbued with this vision asked staff members to submit proposals for new work projects that would express their gifts and passions (Caudron 1997).

A feature of professional life is that one's personhood is indissolubly linked to one's work. What van den Berg (2002) says of teaching applies to the general situation in the other human service professions as well: 'Teachers invest their "selves" in their work, which means that the classroom and/or school become the main sites for the development of self-esteem and self-fulfillment…' (p.586). It is therefore vitally important that the organisational leadership support the professional development of their staff. Moreover, leaders need to act as catalysts on occasion. That is, they need to be searching for creative pathways to self-actualisation to offer staff (Krajewski 1996). To be sure, self-actualisation is a function of individual action. In particular, it is facilitated by perceptive and informed reflection on professional practice (Dodd 2001). However, the leadership also has a role. Rather than wait for staff to complain of boredom and lack of fulfilment, principals and clinical managers need to be continually working on plans with the potential for stimulation of personal and professional growth.

To recapitulate the discussion thus far, if staff members are to feel that they belong in their places of work, they need to have a sense that management is taking their needs, concerns and aspirations seriously. When management hears and responds to their legitimate claims, staff members feel that they have been accorded the status of 'citizenship' in the workplace community. A citizen has rights and privileges, as well as duties and responsibilities. She cannot simply be treated as an object; she is a person whose dignity and worth must be recognised. A 'responsive' work environment generates a sense of citizenship and community.

Identifying with the organisational ethos

Every society has its own particular set of customs, beliefs, values and goals. Over time it has 'cultivated' this pattern of shared meaning, and so we refer to the culture of a particular group of people. A number of social scientists and organisational theorists have observed that firms are actually mini-societies and that it is therefore appropriate to refer to corporate or organisational culture (Kotter and Heskett 1992; McCoy 1985, ch.3; Morgan 1986, ch.5). McCoy (1985) helpfully suggests that a corporate culture is made up of *customs, values* and *purposes*. Customs are those behaviours and rituals which have gained general approval over time and have thus established themselves as social habits within the organisation. Whether or not certain actions and behaviours will be accepted in the course of the organisation's development depends on what standards and norms of evaluation the organisation establishes. That is to say, values have a central role in shaping a corporate culture. Purposes 'express values in terms of goals to be attained in the future' and thus form the basis for change and development within an organisation. 'Taken together, customs, values, and purposes are cohesive elements binding persons and groups into a community' (McCoy 1985, p.64).

Now of course there are often competing desires in relation to the shape of the organisational culture. One common clash is between a vision of success and organisational prestige, on the one hand, and one in which the humanising values of justice, compassion and togetherness are central, on the other. We are taking our lead from covenant theology. In the life of Israel, and later of the church, the ethical quality of relationships was an absolutely central concern. Our preference is for the promotion of humanising cultures. It is really a question of where the emphasis lies. Everyone wants to see his or her organisation succeed. Some are quite ruthless in their pursuit of their goals; others care about people and about the quality of their working relationships. If the level of dissonance is high, the culture will be one of conflict and competition. When the level is low, however, there is an opportunity to work towards a common vision.

Through promoting a particular set of values and purposes the members of the organisation 'enact' a shared reality (Morgan 1986). The values we hold, the purposes we set for ourselves, constitute our interpretative schema. As individuals bring their various interpretative schemas to bear on their organisational life a certain culture is shaped. The upshot of this is that the members of an organisation do not simply find themselves situated in a fixed social reality; they actually engage – sometimes unconsciously – in shaping that reality.

The way different individuals interpret the life of their organisation will, we have noted, be marked by pluralism. Thus, at certain critical points in the development of an organisational culture, there will be collisions between competing interpretative systems.

Let us at this point attend to the significant clashes in interpretative schemas in hospitals and schools. Amongst the professionals with responsibility for care of the sick, there is a division between those who hold up technology and cure as primary, on the one hand, and those who emphasise caring and non-technological interventions, on the other

(Kitson 2001). This, then, is the collision between curing and caring. Both are important, of course. The real question is this: Where is the emphasis to be placed in the shaping of the hospital culture?

The same tension between technological intervention and human support gets played out in midwifery services. In that context, it is referred to in terms of medicalised and humanised birth (Wagner 2002). Guiding the latter vision is the belief that birth is a natural process and the role of the midwife is primarily to support the autonomic responses. Those who adopt a medical model of birthing argue that the technology facilitates safe birthing. The central question in relation to this clash of visions is the locus of control. 'In medicalized birth the doctor is always in control while the key element in humanized birth is the woman in control of her own birthing and whatever happens to her' (Wagner 2002, p.213).

In turning to the educational environment, lastly, we also find differences in relation to the question of school culture. There are those, for example, who value justice, inclusion, mutuality and care (Strachan 1999). Over against such persons, one finds those who are motivated primarily by the goals of excellence in student achievement and high school prestige. This is the clash between a justice vision and an elitist one.

In order for a person to feel that she belongs in her organisation, she needs to be able to identify with the prevailing culture. If a nurse, midwife or teacher finds herself on the wrong side of one of the divides sketched above, she will feel frustrated, angry and depressed. Rather than enjoying the feeling of being at home in her work, she will experience the pain of alienation.

It was a lack of congruence between personal and corporate values which resulted in the 8th century BC prophets feeling estranged from their community. *Torah's* insistence on faithfulness, justice and compassion was being ignored by many. A popular view was that the observance of the ritual requirements of Torah would satisfy Yahweh and ensure Yahweh's blessing. But the prophets knew that what Yahweh required was a communal life animated and inspired by the principles of fidelity, justice and love:

> Stop bringing meaningless offerings! Your incense is detestable to me. New Moons, Sabbaths and convocations – I cannot bear your evil assemblies. Your New Moon festivals and your appointed feasts my soul hates. They have become a burden to me; I am weary of bearing them.

When you spread out your hands in prayer, I will hide my eyes from you; even if you offer many prayers, I will not listen. Your hands are full of blood; wash and make yourselves clean. Take your evil deeds out of my sight! Stop doing wrong, learn to do right!

Seek justice, encourage the oppressed. Defend the cause of the fatherless, plead the case of the widow. (Isa 1:13–17)

The prophets and all those who identified fully with Yahweh's plan would only feel at home in their community if there was a radical change of thought and practice.

The members of the Deuteronomistic movement in the 7th century BC felt the same deep sense of alienation. The particular focus of their concern was on apostasy and the way in which the people had infected themselves with foreign beliefs and practices. As we saw above in our discussion of covenant theology, the theologians in this movement used the stories of the ancestors in their attempt to reshape the culture of Israel. They wanted to re-establish the original values and priorities, namely worship of the one true God and a life of fidelity to *Torah*. Here we see the main features in the background to the new covenant (Jer 31:31–34). In the light of the persistent waywardness of the people, God proposed a radical renovation of the covenant in which God would act miraculously to move fidelity to new heights.

McCoy (1985, pp.184–185) highlights the importance of story-telling in shaping the culture of an organisation. To tell a story is to engage in 'meaning-bearing action'. It is when certain narratives catch hold of the imagination of the members of an organisation that the culture begins to change. I share the vision of those who want to humanise institutions and their practices. What the humanising visions in nursing, midwifery and teaching have in common is a total commitment to the person-centred vision. An important part of the strategy of those who want to change the culture of their organisation is story-telling. They tell the stories that remind others that the individual – the patient, the woman or the student – is ultimately the reason the institution exists. These are the stories that highlight the power in compassion, empathy and self-giving. They are the stories of professional and client sharing the journey for a time and bestowing precious gifts along the way.

For some, it will be a long time before they can feel that they truly belong in their organisation. The prevailing ethos simply does not reflect their core values. Sadly, the wholesome experience of being at home lies in the future. The feeling that many long for is expressed simply and eloquently by M.L. Brownsberger. In reflecting on his professional life, he has this to say: 'To me, the places [of work] supported my person; my person was congruent with my places. My person was organized around an ethic and focused. The ethic was the work; the work was the ethic. I was at home' (Brownsberger 1995, p.667).

In this chapter, our concern has been to explore the relationship between a sense of belonging and psychological well-being. Belonging, we said, is related to appropriate recognition of personhood and of achievement, to responsiveness to legitimate needs and concerns, and to a feeling of ownership of the corporate vision. We have used a number of theological perspectives operating in covenantal life and thought to shape our discussion. Following the biblical line, we developed the following principles. First, recognition of personhood is at least as important as, and probably more important than, recognition of achievements. Second, there is great value in a proactive approach to promoting the well-being of employees. Third, the needs of those most at risk need to be given priority. And lastly, people need a good and right vision with which to align themselves if they are to feel at home.

In the next chapter, we will reflect on the important issue of trust in workplace relations, and again we will use covenant theology to inform the analysis. We have observed in this chapter that identification with a vision is of central importance in the life of an organisation. This will be developed further in what follows.

CHAPTER 6

Trust in the Organisation

More and more, trust is being identified as a vital element in effective organisations. If working relationships are to be effective, high levels of communication and co-operation are required. Trust is the 'lubricant' that enables workplace operations to flow smoothly. When people have confidence in each other's words and deeds the level of friction is very low or non-existent.

In general, both management and staff value trust in the workplace. Managers view trust, as they do everything else, primarily in terms of efficiency. They recognise that the smooth running of the organisation is enhanced through a trust-based environment. Trust reduces uncertainty about the future and the necessity for continually guarding against opportunistic behaviour. It allows for fluent, harmonious organisational functioning by eliminating friction and minimising the need for bureaucratic structures which monitor behaviour. On the whole, employees also acknowledge the importance of trust. On the one hand, they want to be able to trust that management has their best interests at heart and shares their values. On the other hand, they generally appreciate being trusted. When they are given responsibility and monitoring is minimised they feel valued as employees and as persons. Moreover, when they are entrusted with a high level of self-direction and self-control they have an opportunity to express creativity.

These considerations point to the pastoral implications of trust in the organisation. A trust-based work environment produces a sense of well-being and enhances job satisfaction. When managers feel confident that staff members are committed to organisational goals and will perform their tasks accordingly, a considerable source of stress is removed. Staff members also benefit. While an increased level of responsibility and expectation brings a certain stress, it is a positive one. Both challenge and satisfaction come with being afforded significant levels of autonomy and participation in decision making.

In this chapter, this vitally important issue of trust in organisational life will be viewed through the lens of covenant theology. I will be endeavouring to show how the covenant theme informs and illuminates the discussion of trust taking place amongst organisational theorists. It is not immediately obvious that a relationship between God and God's people in a cultural setting far removed from that in which the issue of labour relations is worked out could speak in any meaningful way to that issue. In order to show that there is in fact a strong connection, I will seek to demonstrate that *partnership* is an appropriate link term. A partnership is built through dialogue. Dialogue, in turn, has at least two basic requirements. First, the parties must be able to include themselves in each other's aims, needs and aspirations. That is, each partner must be able to imaginatively experience reality from the side of the other. Second, there must be a commitment to work with the other in achieving her legitimate aims. My argument will be that in the covenant relationship with Israel, and later with all people, God has established an ideal for these two essential characteristics in dialogue.

The dialogical process aimed at mutual understanding and, beyond that, at working together cannot be established without high levels of trust. Trust is clearly an essential ingredient in a strong partnership. Genuine dialogue involves a movement beyond trust based on monitoring and control ('deterrence-based trust'), beyond even that which is associated with knowledge and the ability to predict the behaviour of the other ('knowledge-based trust'), to trust which is established through *identification* (Shapiro *et al.* 1992). The highest form of trust is that which comes when the preferences of the other have been internalised. God's deepest intention in establishing the covenant, as we saw in the last chapter, is for the people to internalise the divine will and purpose. While the Decalogue was written on tablets of stone, God intended that the people would take it into their hearts. The ideal of identification between God and the people reached a high point in the new covenant proclaimed by the 7th and 6th century BC prophets and ultimately fulfilled in Christ. The partnership between God and Israel, and later between Christ and the church, demonstrates, I will be suggesting, in a most vivid way a fact which social psychologists and organisational theorists have been recently establishing through empirical research. That fact is that when there is a strong sense of group identity persons tend to own the corporate vision.

The chapter is structured as follows. First, I will attempt to show that partnership is in fact an appropriate covenant rubric. Next, I will analyse contemporary management–employee relations. The shape of this partnership will then be interpreted with reference to covenant realities. Finally, I will analyse identification-based trust in the light of the covenant and apply the principles developed to the particular case of human service organisations.

Partnership as the link between the covenant and management–employee relations

Others have also endeavoured to use the theology of the covenant as an interpretative tool in analysing relationships in an organisation. For example, the Christian business ethicist Stewart Herman argues that *vulnerability* is the rubric which links covenant thinking with the realties of the management–employee relationship (Herman 1995, 1997). However, I believe that the way he uses the term 'vulnerability' in relation to the covenant is problematical. I want to discuss his approach briefly before outlining my own.

Herman (1997, p.32) suggests that contingency, risk and vulnerability are key terms in a covenant ethic, and that as these factors are also crucial in management–employee relations the possibility of covenant theology informing organisational theory is indicated. Consider, first, the situation in the workplace. Employees, on one side, are vulnerable because they may be forced to cope with underpayment, excessive workload, unsatisfactory and/or unsafe conditions, and even dismissal. On the other side, management is vulnerable to 'costs' imposed by labour. Examples of these costs are organised resistance, lack of care, less than optimal effort, absenteeism and sabotage.

In the covenant relationship, Herman observes, there is also a mutual vulnerability. God's vulnerability, first, is associated with the divine 'project'. The aim in this project is 'to fashion the people of Israel, and later the church, into a moral community faithful to God alone' (Herman 1997, p.45). This goal, suggests Herman (1997), 'renders God vulnerable to the failure of the people to respond appropriately' (p.45). While the people certainly do for extended periods act wisely, courageously and loyally, all too often they fall into forgetfulness, waywardness and rebellion. In the covenant relationship the people are also vulnerable. They seek deliverance from infertility, landlessness, lawlessness and enemies, but God 'is anything but a reliable tool of their desires, anything but a powerful provider molded in their image' (Herman 1997, p.45). While God stands always ready to bless, God is quick to chastise when it is required. Indeed, there is always the threat of the ultimate curses: abandonment and even destruction.

While it is evident that vulnerability is a central factor in relations between management and employees, it is not so clear that it is an appropriate rubric to apply to covenant relations. Certainly the people of Israel were vulnerable to divine chastisement. The covenant promises carry with them the threat of curse if Israel is unfaithful. But I contend that it is inappropriate to highlight judgement through selecting vulnerability as a covenant metaphor. The *primary* aim in God's relationship with Israel is God's gracious self-communication through acts of protection, provision and deliverance. Divine chastisement is aimed at keeping Israel in that spiritual condition which allows the bestowal of blessings. The curse of the covenant has a very definite role, but it is a subsidiary one. In using the covenant to interpret vertical workplace relations it seems odd to make a connection via a sub- rather than a superordinate principle. Moreover, what is really striking about early Israel's perception of its situation is that it is characterised not by a sense of vulnerability but of confidence and hope (Bright 1979). (See, for example, The Oracles of Balaam [Num 23–24]; The Blessing of Moses [Deut 33]; The Blessing of Jacob [Gen 49]; The Song of Miriam [Ex 15:1–18]; and The Song of Deborah [Jdg 5].) An extract from Moses' Blessing gives the flavour of this confident view of the nation's future prospects:

> The eternal God is your refuge, and underneath are the everlasting arms. He will drive out your enemy before you, saying, 'Destroy him!' So Israel will live in safety alone; Jacob's spring is secure in a land of grain and new wine where the heavens drop dew. Blessed are you, O Israel! Who is like you, a people saved by the Lord? He is your shield and helper and your glorious sword. Your enemies will cower before you, and you will trample down their high places. (Deut 33:27–29)

When one considers early Israel's actual situation, this positive, hopeful outlook is hard to credit. It had neither great military strength nor material security. The reality was a loose confederation of tribes, poorly armed, operating without a central authority, and continually under threat of attack. The land was not rich and fertile – far from it. It was quite difficult to satisfy the bodily needs of the people. In the face of these imposing difficulties and threats to well-being, the earliest Israelites were hopeful because they remembered the God who had covenanted for sure protection and abundant provision. They felt vulnerable to poor soil, unfavourable weather and enemy invasion, but confident that Yahweh would transform the distress of the present into a glorious future. The covenant, far from being orientated to mistrust and vulnerability, was an instrument used by God to instil a sense of assurance. As Most (1967) observes, this was particularly important in light of the fact that Israel found itself in an environment in which people felt vulnerable before their deities:

> Human beings in general are apt to mistrust God, saying: His ways are above ours as the heavens are above the earth: Who can understand them? Israel in particular came from a milieu in which the gods were the object of mistrust. A covenant could be a device of love to make [people] know where they stand, to reassure them that at least under specified conditions they may have confidence. (p.7)

If the use of vulnerability to characterise the people's situation in the covenant is problematic, its use with reference to the divine involvement is even more so. How, I want to ask, can the notion that God is vulnerable to the people be squared with the doctrine of divine sovereignty? To suggest that the people's waywardness renders God vulnerable to frustration in the divine project of fashioning a moral and faithful community implies that God is somehow in a position of reliance. This is hardly the biblical view: 'Can a man be of benefit to God? Can even a wise man benefit him? What pleasure would it give the Almighty if you were righteous? What would he gain if your ways were blameless?' (Job 22:23). Actually, God's purpose and plan is broader than Herman indicates. In moulding a moral community, God's ultimate aim is for Israel to be 'a light to the nations' (Isa 49:6). God uses the chosen people as a witness so that the nations may know God and the offer of salvation, and constantly calls them, God's people, to fidelity in service of the divine purposes. But ultimately God does not rely on them. Walton (1994) makes the following apt comment:

> God's revelatory objectives can be achieved with or without Israel's help. If they cooperate, there is benefit for them. If they fail there is punishment. God's program is never in jeopardy... (p.52)

God used the people of Israel as a witness to the nations and formed them in the divine way in order to strengthen the testimony. When the people were wayward the witness was weakened, but that did not mean that Israel had the power to ultimately frustrate God's project.

Given that there seem to be insurmountable problems associated with the choice of vulnerability as a term linking the covenant and management–employee relations, it is necessary to find a more appropriate one. Whatever rubric one chooses it is not possible, of course, to set up a perfect match between the two sets of relational realities. Nevertheless, the metaphor should at least connect with a central aspect of the covenant, on the one hand, and have within it the potential for illuminating the vertical workplace relationship, on the other. With this in mind, I suggest *partnership* as the connecting term. A genuine partnership is built on trust, and trust, in turn, is established in dialogue. We will have to interpret the dialogue between God and Israel carefully, however. It does not parallel exactly the ideal for communication in the contemporary workplace. Whereas modern workers demand equal status and power symmetry in pressing their demands, Israel's pleas and protests could ultimately be put only as prayer. That it was nevertheless a real dialogue is due to God's grace, solicitude and absolute commitment to the people's well-being. Here, I suggest, is the point at which the style of partnership expressed in the covenant can speak to the management–employee relationship. While words such as 'grace', 'mercy' and 'lovingkindness' may not connect with the hard realities of industrial relations, the divine commitment to understand the concerns of Israel and to work vigourously for its welfare surely does. The first task, however, if we are to use the idea of partnership, is to show that it is an appropriate covenant rubric.

Partnership as a covenant rubric

In the last chapter, I referred at one point to the covenant partnership between Yahweh and Israel. While theologians tend to use this language quite freely, we need to acknowledge that there is a good deal of debate in the biblical studies field over whether the term 'partnership' is entirely appropriate. There are some scholars of the Hebrew Scriptures who argue that the covenant between God and Israel is unilateral in nature.[1] There is on this view no sense of an agreement involving equal partners. In the *berith* with Israel God has the sole initiative. God declares God's promises to the people, on the one hand, and lays down the obligations associated with those promises, on the other. Thus, Yahweh comes to Israel in a twofold way: through grace and with the law. It is not difficult to find a theological reason why some scholars would feel disinclined to construe the covenant in terms of partnership. If the notion of a bilateral relationship between Yahweh and Israel is projected, the doctrine of divine grace and sovereignty seems to be contradicted. While I can readily agree that the initiative in the covenant relationship is clearly with God and that the people do not stand on an equal footing with God, I still want to argue that there is a biblical warrant for the idea of a partnership. Here I am guided by Nicholson's (1986) interpretation. He argues that the bilateral nature of the covenant can be established through a reference to what is probably the earliest description of the making of such a covenant, which is Ex 24:3–8. Here there is certainly an emphasis on Israel's obligation *vis-à-vis* the commandments, but the pledge of obedience to the commandments is related to a ceremony which effected a solemn consecration of Israel as Yahweh's holy people. It is not solely a question of God announcing the divine promises and imposing obligations on the people. There are obligations, but there is also *fellowship.*

Those who characterise the covenant as unilateral in nature fail, Nicholson contends, to take sufficient note of the fact that Israel had to choose and to decide. The covenant represents on the one hand the great promises of Yahweh concerning Israel's destiny and role among the nations. These promises, however, are not unconditional. If the people are to receive the blessings God has pledged, they must respond to God's invitation through declaring and actualising their commitment. That is to say, the making and the keeping of the covenant involved a choosing and deciding on Israel's part over time. At Sinai Israel chose to enter the covenant. On two occasions the people responded to Moses' reading of the commandments with a commitment to fidelity (Ex 24:3–8). On the plains of Moab the next generation chose and declared that 'this day' Yahweh had become its God (Deut 26:17).

Everything in the covenant did not begin and end with the divine actions, though they were certainly primary. The people needed to choose and decide, to declare their commitment to participate in Yahweh's project. With this data before him, Nicholson (1986) considers it appropriate to refer to the covenant in terms of partnership and fellowship:

> The making of the covenant was not only upon Yahweh's initiative; more than that, he himself was a partner to it. In no sense, therefore, did the covenant theology conceive of life as mere observance, upon penalty of disaster, of divinely decreed laws. Rather, life for Israel was understood as fellowship with Yahweh who had entered a covenant with this people, and the fulfilment of Yahweh's commandments was to be an expression of this fellowship. (p.215)

This partnership between Yahweh and Israel clearly had a goal and an objective. There is debate amongst Hebrew Scripture scholars as to whether the term which primarily expresses the purpose of the covenant is redemption (Most 1967; von Rad 1975), relationship (Vriezen 1970) or revelation (Walton 1994). For our purposes, it is sufficient to simply observe that the three are indissolubly linked together. The Hebrew Scriptures tell a story of God at work in the world revealing the divine self – its nature, will and purpose – in order that Israel first, and then all peoples, might enter into a redemptive relationship. The covenant is a device God used to facilitate God's programme of revelation and redemption.

The partnership between management and employees is, of course, orientated to quite different goals and objectives. It is appropriate to connect covenant and the employment relation, nevertheless, because both partnerships involve the same general principle. Both in the Hebrew Scriptures and in the contemporary workplace we find two parties working together in pursuit of a common goal. Or at least this was then, and is today, the ideal. Sometimes the people of Israel all but lost sight of where God was leading them. And all too often the goal of achieving constructive working relations is thwarted by mistrust, power asymmetry and opportunism.

The partnership between management and employees

A covenant between two parties is built on mutual trust. The organisational theorists Creed and Miles (1996) contend that managerial assumptions and expectations are the key factors in building trust within the organisation: 'Managerial philosophies,' they write, 'are the mechanisms that serve to focus expectations about people and so shape trust in organizations' (p.20). It is true that management must take a lead; however, I will be suggesting that trust is built up in a dialogue between the two partners. Staff members have their own particular perspectives, values and areas of expertise. Unless this fact is taken seriously there can never be a genuine partnership. A partnership is founded on, and strengthened by, dialogue. Dialogue requires a willingness both to include oneself in, and to commit oneself to, the legitimate aims and aspirations of the other. Put simply, the parties must be ready to listen and to act. The first step is an imaginative entry into the concerns and hopes of the other. If the dialogue is to be ongoing, beyond openness to the other party's appeals there must be a committed follow-up on the agreements made. Concerned listening and fidelity to pledges are, it goes without saying, basic requirements if there is to be trust. Dialogue needs trust as a platform to build on; and to the extent that the dialogue is successful, trust grows stronger.

Keeping in mind the fact that trust is a dialogical reality, it is still true that managerial philosophy is a critical factor in the process. The analysis by Creed and Miles (1996) shows how the moves from the traditional understanding of labour (the 19th century), through the human relations approach (early 1900s to early 1950s), to the current human resources model have increasingly tended to engender trust. The traditional model was conditioned by social Darwinist thinking. On this view, there is in the economic sphere, as elsewhere, a 'natural law' at work, according to which the fit survive and the unfit perish.[2] A 'fit' business is one in which managers are able to elicit from a generally unwilling workforce optimal effort through close control. Workers perceive work as a burden, and in order to get the best from them it is necessary for management to be both vigilant and firm.

In the human relations model, by contrast, there is an appreciation of basic human aspirations. As I suggested in the previous chapter, people want to belong and they need to be recognised both as employees and as persons. And as Fukuyama (1995) observes, there is ample empirical evidence for such a view:

> [W]orkers do not want to be treated like cogs in a large machine, isolated from managers and fellow workers, with little pride in their skills or their organization, and trusted with a minimal amount of authority and control over the work they do for a living. Any number of empirical studies from Elton Mayo on have indicated that workers are happier in group-oriented organizations than in more individualistic ones. (pp.355–356)

Belonging and recognition, then, are key terms in the human relations model. Workers value both a group identity and individual acknowledgement.

In the human resources philosophy, these two fundamental human aspirations are recognised. But there is a particular stress on two other factors, namely participation and creativity. Most people, it is assumed, want to be involved in organisational goal setting, are ready to assume responsibility, and are looking for opportunities for self-expression. (Actually, as I argued in the last chapter, the four principles are interrelated. Workers feel a sense of belonging, feel that their value as persons is recognised, when they are encouraged to participate in decision making and contribute to product and service innovation. What separates the two philosophies is the place at which the emphasis is put.) On this human resources view, the workforce has an untapped potential which must be utilised if the organisation is to make gains in productivity.

It is evident that in this progression in managerial thinking which began with a pessimistic assessment of worker motivation and capability and has ended in a recognition of the (general) desire for participation and responsibility, the potential for trust-building has dramatically increased. At the turn of the century there was a gulf dividing management and labour. Authoritarianism and lack of respect on the part of the former, and fear and suspicion in the ranks of the latter, meant that the idea of a partnership was nowhere to be seen. As soon as the executive sector began, however, to recognise employees' needs for belonging, recognition and participation, the workplace relationship started to move in the direction of mutuality and co-operation.

In schools and hospitals, an important area in which the move to mutuality and co-operation has found expression is in collaborative decision making. Ray and Turkel (2002) observe that trust in health care organisations is created when practising nurses and administrators work together on organisational decisions. The authors acknowledge that nurses believe that they have vital knowledge to contribute and want to be seen as equal partners in the management process. Tschannen-Moran and Hoy (2000), in referring to the school context, make the same observation concerning practitioner knowledge being valued. They contend that the school administration must have a sincere expectation that teachers will provide important insights for genuine collaboration to take place. This genuine collaboration is contrasted with a contrived one in which teachers are involved in decision making merely as a gesture towards the new human resources approach. The aim is not the building of a trust-based organisation, but rather to keep teachers 'happy' and loyal.

The human resources philosophy, I have been saying, works with the premise that employees do, on the whole, aspire to participation, autonomy and creative self-expression. In an article aimed at the description of a normative view of work, Mückenberger (1996) employs the suggestive metaphor of 'citizenship' to capture these desiderata. Citizens, he notes, recognise each other as equals. In this relation of mutuality an individual is able to communicate her concerns, interests and aims. When two people or two parties communicate in the full sense, Mückenberger suggests, there is dialogue, and out of dialogue community is formed. Necessarily associated with equality and communal sharing is a recognition of rights. Any note of authoritarianism, any thought of employee dependency, must be eschewed by management. Rather, there needs to be a full recognition of employee rights. These include the right (a) to organise their own lives, including their time; (b) to have access to education, training and periods of leave; (c) to refuse work that is potentially harmful either to them personally, to the society at large, or to the environment; (d) of women to full and equal participation; and (e) to shape work to mesh with parenting responsibilities (for example, in Sweden wage compensation is provided as an incentive to share the parenting role). These, then, are the principal rights of a citizen in the workplace. For worker citizenship to become a reality, however, there needs to be dialogue that is grounded in trust: 'The underlying aim of all these proposals is to develop in the wage employment sphere a form of dialogue based on genuine communication, on freely consented coordination and mutual trust' (Mückenberger 1996, p.687).

Unfortunately, the conditions for trust in the dialogue are too often absent. Each social actor, observes Mückenberger, tends to de-emphasise or even discount the values and aims of the others. There is a proclivity for judging the preferences of others as incomprehensible and irrational. When this happens, a dynamic of 'mutual obstructionism' (Mückenberger 1996, p.688) is set up. Good will is almost entirely absent and a power struggle develops which makes dialogue impossible. What is required is a movement beyond obstructionism to a 'modern and intelligent approach to conflict resolution' (Mückenberger 1996, p.689). In this dialogue and consultation, there is the creation of the conditions for mutual recognition of aims, interests and values.

This mutual recognition, as we saw in Chapter 1, is what Buber calls 'inclusion'. Recall that it involves 'the extension of one's own concreteness, the fulfilment of the actual situation of life, the complete presence of the reality in which one participates' (Buber 1947, p.97). In order to include oneself in the reality of the other, one must be able to imaginatively 'swing' into his way of engaging with others, work and the society. The failure of dialogue, when it comes, comes because one or both parties have not been able to grasp the preferences of the other. In the absence of any real receptivity to the fears, hopes and values of the other party, there is a fall into monologue, with all of its unwholesome and ultimately destructive possibilities. If there is to be a partnership between the two sectors in the employment sphere, one which is based on a recognition of the citizenship of the employee on the one side and on a commitment to contribute optimally to productivity on the other, there needs to be genuine communication and a dialogical relation. Without inclusion there is no basis for workplace dialogue.

Something which Mückenberger does not address directly, but which is implied in his analysis, is the fact that the trust which is foundational in dialogue can only be established when the parties have previously demonstrated fidelity to pledges made. Beyond the rhetoric of agreements there needs to be committed action. There is what some have called 'instrumental' or 'strategic' ethics in the commercial world (Quinn and Jones 1995). In this approach to employment and business, there is a belief that it is possible to use others to achieve goals by acting with just enough integrity to convince others that one really does have integrity. The obvious problem with this policy is that sooner or later one will be found out. If the plan is to operate with only minimum levels of openness, flexibility and respect, to do just enough to convince the other party to contribute to one's programme, one is on very shaky dialogical ground. The other will soon enough become aware that integrity is lacking and any trust that was there will be shattered. Rhetoric and posturing, with a sprinkling of actions in support of pledges offered, cannot for long be passed off as commitment and integrity. The latter qualities are what is required to produce an environment of trust, communication and co-operation.

The organisational partnership in a covenantal perspective

Above we have considered the general conditions for the establishment of trust and co-operation between management and employees. In a modern and intelligent interpretation of work, there is recognition of the legitimacy of, and value in, employee participation and autonomy. Is it now possible to contribute something new to this contemporary definition of the employment relation through a theological analysis? More specifically, we need to ask the question: What illumination can the theology of the covenant provide? It will be immediately obvious that there are constraints on how far the parallel between covenant thinking and a modern reading of the work situation can be extended. In the employment relationship the ideal is equality between the partners. That is, there is symmetry in the power relations. But in the covenant partnership the humans are not full partners in the sense that they are entitled to assume equal responsibility with God in determining the project which shapes their life and destiny. As Vriezen (1970) puts it:

> The discussion between God and [the human] is never a dialogue pure and simple; the [human] who speaks must always realize and experience that he is addressing himself to the *Holy One*, and his word or answer spoken to God can fundamentally be a prayer only. (p.160)

Despite the fact that there is a gap between covenant theology and the employment relation, I suggest that the former does in fact have within it the capacity to inform our understanding of the latter. The theology of the covenant does this by providing an ideal to which both parties in the workplace partnership should aspire. There are, as we have seen, two basic conditions for dialogue in the employment sphere. The first is that the parties must include themselves in each other's concerns and aspirations. Fidelity to pledges is the second. It is in relation to these two conditions that the divine participation in the covenant partnership sets the standard.

In the Hebrew Scriptures, divine transcendence is emphasised. It is not possible, in Israel's world, to look upon the divine visage and live. God reveals Godself through a series of theophanies. In the burning bush, in the lightning, thunder and smoke, God is present to the people. The absolute holiness of God establishes this distance from God's creatures. And yet, God comes very near in loving concern. God meets with the people at a distance, but at the same time draws near to them in their suffering and distress. At the scene of the burning bush Yahweh refers to a 'coming down' to deliver the Hebrew slaves:

> I have indeed seen the misery of my people in Egypt. I have heard them crying out because of their slave drivers, and I am concerned about their suffering. So I have come down to rescue them from the hand of the Egyptians and to bring them up out of that land into a good and spacious land, a land flowing with milk and honey... (Exod 3:7–8)

God took into the divine heart the aspirations of the slave people for freedom, land and a prosperous and enjoyable life.

At the time of the Babylonian Exile the people were in a state of deep mourning and despair. They had experienced the ultimate disaster, which was the loss of their homeland. Naturally they thought that their God had forgotten them. It seemed as though God's loving concern had all but evaporated. God reassured the people with these beautiful words:

> Can a mother forget the baby at her breast and have no compassion on the child she has borne? Though she may forget, I will not forget you! See, I have engraved you on the palms of my hands; your walls are ever before me. (Isa 49:15–16)

The image of mother and child is suggestive in relation to inclusion. The needs of the infant are constantly before the mother. She cannot afford to ignore them even for a short time. Moreover, she needs to imaginatively grasp the reality of her child if she is to give the help and care that is required. Lacking the facility of speech, the baby cannot communicate precisely what she needs from her mother. It is the mother's capacity to understand her baby's situation which fills in the missing information. In one sense the tender love of a mother for her child is an engagement very far removed from the hard realities of workplace relationships (there is a similar gap in relation to the harsh realities of the divine chastisement associated with the covenant). When, however, the metaphor is seen as pointing to a desire to enter fully into the needs, concerns and hopes of the other, it has something very significant to say in the context of organisational life. Management needs to put itself in the staff's position, to engage, for example, with their anxiety when they talk about work overload and/or job insecurity, or with their frustration when they talk about external directives conflicting with their own values and preferences. On the other hand, staff members need to be able to imaginatively swing into management's reality. They might, for instance, connect with the strain of trying to balance diverse and often competing expectations, or with the pressure that is associated with being ultimately responsible for the organisation's effectiveness.

When it comes to the new covenant in Christ, God's inclusion of Godself in the realities of human existence reaches the apogee. The bearer of the final covenant of salvation is the God-person. Once it was 'in the spirit' that God engaged with the realities of human existence; now the engagement is in the flesh. 'Incarnation represents the possibility of crossing over fully, of genuinely entering another world' (McCarthy 1992, p.128). Here, then, is another rich and evocative metaphor for inclusion. The two images – mothering and incarnation – are suggestive of a strong commitment to experience life from the other side. It is this swing into the other's realities which is essential if there is to be a movement in management–staff relationship beyond 'mutual obstructionism' to constructive dialogue.

It is interesting to note at this point that observers of both the school and the hospital environment find that inclusion is facilitated through leader visibility (Krajewski 1996; Ray and Turkel 2002; Tschannen-Moran and Hoy 2000). Krajewski (1996) makes reference to a principal who was regularly seen in the classrooms, the lounge and the library. He thought of the entire school as his office. Similarly, the nursing administrator needs to make the wards her office. In making rounds with staff, the administrator is able to 'walk in their shoes'. She puts herself in the best place for connecting with the realities of her staff.

Dialogue, as we have observed, needs also a backdrop of fidelity to pledges if it is to be successful. If either party has in the past demonstrated an unwillingness to honour commitments there is no platform of trust on which to build constructive communication. It is Yahweh's fidelity in the covenant relationship which presents as an ideal for the partnership between management and labour. If the former relationship really is a partnership, as I have argued that it is, it must be bilateral in nature. Most (1967) suggests that it is bilateral in the sense (at least) that both God and the people take on obligations. A question that he is primarily interested in in his discussion is why it was that God kept to God's commitments. It cannot be that God owes the people anything. The obvious answer is that it was the divine righteousness which bound God in the covenant. It is interesting and instructive to follow Most as he expands on this answer. In the psalms there are appeals to the covenant bond, *chesed* (mercy, lovingkindness): 'Turn, O Lord, and deliver me; save me because of your *chesed*' (Ps 6:4). We also find pleas based on God's *sedaqah* (righteousness): 'In you, O Lord, I have taken refuge; let me never be put to shame. Rescue me and deliver me in your sedaqah' (Ps 71:1–2). As these appeals, Most points out, seem parallel to the appeals to the covenant, it appears that for Yahweh to dispense mercy is a matter of righteousness. Indeed, this possibility is confirmed through a reference to a number of psalms in which mercy and righteousness are intimately linked: 'Continue your mercy to those who know you, your *righteousness* to the upright of heart' (Ps 36:10). And similarly: 'For your name's sake, O Lord, preserve my life; in your *righteousness*, bring me out of trouble. In your *mercy*, silence my enemies, destroy all my foes, for I am your servant' (Ps 143:11–12). Most (1967) concludes that 'God's exercise of *chesed* is considered to be an exercise of *sedaqah*. That is, for him to keep his part under the covenant, is a matter of moral righteousness. Hence, he must have bound himself' (p.5).

God's commitment to the covenant is a question of moral integrity. To the cause of Israel's liberty, peace and prosperity, Yahweh was totally committed. Owing nothing to the people, God bound Godself as a matter of *sedaqah*. The term 'integrity' rather than 'righteousness', it goes without saying, fits the context of industrial relations. In the covenant relationship God displayed time and again God's integrity, fidelity and total commitment to the people. Though they at different times fell into waywardness and rebellion, in their better moments they knew that they could trust in, and rely on, Yahweh. It is this divine integrity and fidelity which I am upholding as the standard for the dialogical relations between management and staff.

When inclusion and integrity are demonstrated there is a readiness to trust. Trust is foundational in any workplace partnership. It can and does, however, take different forms. Trust in an organisation is not always at the level produced through empathy and moral uprightness. Sometimes it is simply based on control and deterrence. In between is the trust which comes with relational information and a capacity to predict the behaviour of the other party.

Three types of trust in the organisation

Shapiro *et al.* (1992) posit three forms of trust which are common in the business world: deterrence-based, knowledge-based and identification-based trust. Their main interest is in inter-firm relationships. It is quite possible, however, to modify their analysis to fit the management–employee relationship.

The lowest level form of trust in the world of enterprise is that which is based on *deterrence*. We tend to trust others to keep their word when we know that there are constraints on them acting opportunistically. For example, a manager is confident that workers will arrive on time because late arrivers have their pay docked. If deterrence is to establish reliability the impact of the negative consequences of uncooperative behaviour must be judged to be greater than the potential gain through that behaviour. For instance, an employee might choose a pattern of a lie-in and a leisurely breakfast over being on time if she will only have to endure a stern word from time to time, but not if she knows that she will have to ultimately suffer a significant deduction from her pay. The ultimate deterrent is, of course, dismissal. In the contemporary industrial relations climate, however, the grounds for terminating employment are quite tightly defined. It is nevertheless true that most employees value having a job sufficiently that they will at least work to minimally acceptable standards.

Knowledge-based trust is linked to predictability and dependability. In establishing a working relationship, the partners get to know how each other thinks and acts. Over time, for example, a chief executive observes the pattern of a particular manager down the line always completing reports in a timely fashion. She plans her schedule accordingly. If, on the other hand, another manager has demonstrated a tendency to be tardy, trust becomes problematic. Actually, Shapiro *et al.* (1992) argue that even in this situation, trust can result. While they admit that it may seem out of place to speak of trust in relation to uncooperative behaviour, they contend that trust, at its core, 'is simply dependability' (p.369). Being able to predict less than desirable actions renders those actions trustworthy. Such a paradoxical formulation I find unhelpful. An expression such as 'trusting a person to be unreliable' is contrary to our ordinary way of speaking and thinking. Further, it is usually the case that employees and business partners act in an uncooperative way sometimes, but on other occasions their actions meet expectations. If a manager, to return to the example used above, is usually late but sometimes excels himself and turns in the report on time, how is it possible to depend on him to be either late or on schedule? It is far better when talking about trust, I suggest, to refer predictability exclusively to co-operative behaviour.

Identification-based trust is the highest form of trust. It is the kind of trust that is established when the partners internalise each other's preferences. When values are shared and there is a shared sense of interdependence there is no need for monitoring and, consequently, a very high level of confidence that the actions of the other party will accord in every instance with the common vision. It is true that to reach the point of identification a much higher level of investment in the relationship is required than to establish the conditions for the lower levels of trust. However, the benefits are also much greater. One such benefit is that agency becomes a possibility. 'Increased identification enables one to "think like" the other, "feel like" the other, and "respond like" the other' (Lewicki and Bunker 1996, p.123). When an employee has identified with managerial preferences in this way she can be given authority. Where there is an absence of entrusted delegation, on the other hand, inefficiencies will result. Shapiro *et al.* (1992, p.373) give the example of a company which was experiencing problems with its new system of strategically targeted teams. One such team was tying up an inordinate amount of team-member time through the practice of including all members in presentations to senior management and client groups. The reason for involving everyone at all sessions, they discovered, was that it was considered that not all members had identified with the team's and other members' interests.

There was consequently not sufficient trust to delegate a presentation to two or three members.

A second major benefit associated with identification is that it is possible to work in concert in achieving shared goals. As long as management and employees are pursuing their own independent agendas there is no possibility of a shared strategic focus. If, however, the parties are able to take on each other's preferences and, through dialogue, find a suitable strategic plan, they will be able to move efficiently in the direction of their common goals.

Identification in the organisation in the light of the covenant

The sharing of values and a common vision is vitally important in building trust in an organisation. People give of their best when they feel that the vision sponsored by their organisation is worthy, one that they can believe in and own. When this is the case, they will happily contribute their gifts, their energy and their ideas to the flourishing of the organisation. Further, working relationships are stronger and more resilient. In the workplace there are inevitably misunderstandings and disagreements which put a strain on relations. Relationships based on internalisation are able to stand greater stresses than those based on either deterrence or knowledge (Lewicki and Bunker 1996). With identification between two persons comes greater certainty, reliability and relational strength. In a weakly established relationship, there is not the openness and commitment to admit mistakes, to discuss problems and differences. An act which might result in the breakdown of some relationships becomes in an identification-based one an occasion for dialogue and, ultimately, for the strengthening of the bond.

It is generally accepted that internalisation at all levels of an organisation's vision is required if it is to be fully actualised. I want to argue that this process of internalisation is paralleled in a striking way in the covenanting relationship between Yahweh and Israel. Indeed, as we saw in the previous chapter, the intention on God's part was always for the internalisation of the divine instruction. This is not, perhaps, so clear in the Mosaic covenant where the laws are written on tablets of stone and there is a strong emphasis on deterrence (the covenant curses). Nevertheless, what Yahweh demanded of the people was that they take *Torah* into their hearts.

In the new covenant, God would guarantee the writing of the instruction on the hearts of the people through direct action.

The new covenant Jeremiah announced was not like the old 'because they broke my covenant though I was a husband to them' (31:32). In the new era God will put God's law in their minds and write it on their hearts (31:33). This is a description of the complete internalisation of the divine will under the influence of grace. The experience of God in God's dealings with Israel led to the point at which an internalisation of the divine vision was necessary in order to set the divine project on a more secure footing. Because the old covenant was repeatedly broken, the new is necessary. God will shape new persons, persons who identify fully with God's ways because of the miraculous change in them. A strong and reliable partnership, the long experience of covenanting in the life of Israel teaches, requires identification.

The new covenant is established in all its fullness in the salvific action of Christ. Here, too, internalisation is absolutely central. Echoing Jeremiah, Paul tells us that the spirit of Christ writes 'the law of the Spirit of life' in the Christian (Rms 8:2). Indeed, 'if anyone does not have the Spirit of Christ, he does not belong to Christ' (Rms 8:9b).

As the law of Yahweh, and subsequently the law of Christ, was internalised, persons had a profound sense of belonging. To belong means living faithful to the shared vision of the People of God. I suggest that the long history of covenant relations, involving first Israel and later the church, confirms in a most striking way what organisational theorists (Shapiro *et al.* 1992; Shepphard and Tuchinsky 1996; Tsai and Ghosal 1998) and social psychologists (Kramer and Brewer 1984) have established through empirical research. And that is the fact that a strong group identity means that individuals are less likely to draw sharp distinctions between their own interests and the interests of the collective. The biblical experience of the covenanting process underlines the necessity of deepening the relationship between management and staff to the point where a group identity forms.

There is no doubt that an organisation flourishes when there is identification at all levels with a corporate vision. This is often, of course, quite difficult to achieve. Here again there is a parallel with covenant experience. On numerous occasions the people strayed off the path God had pointed out. The vision was most worthy; in their frailty, the people walked away from it. What we saw in the last chapter, however, is that there are those human service professionals who do not consider the organisation's vision to be a worthy one. Those who value caring and relationality, for example, are convinced that this side of patient care is getting lost in their hospital's focus on technology and cure. Or think of a group of midwives committed to a humanised view of birth who find themselves constantly confronted with the medicalised model. Or it may be, finally, that certain teachers with a vision for justice and inclusivity feel that the principal and others in the administration are driven by an overweening concern for the prestige and status of the school. When these kinds of scenarios are played out, the building of trust is problematic. What is required is an honest, intelligent and courageous dialogue concerning the differences in values. The principles for this dialogue we developed more fully above.

What I have been promoting throughout is a humanising vision of organisational life and practice. By a 'humanising' vision, I mean one that places people at the centre of the organisation's life. It is a vision reflected in the mission statements of many schools and hospitals. The welfare of the client is established as the central focus and priorities are set accordingly. A humanising vision also means that all members of the organisation are valued and treated with fairness and respect. The ideals of justice and care permeate the school or the hospital.

It is one thing to have a mission statement affirming a humanising vision; it is quite another for it to be internalised across the organisation. Every member of the hospital or school community has the responsibility of promoting the vision. While every member has a role to play, the administration must take a lead. Here the moral integrity of the leaders is vitally important. This is supported by the research literature. Ray and Turkel (2002) discuss the importance of a 'caring nursing administrator' to a hospital's life. She or he is a 'statesperson' who embodies the principles of goodness, integrity, truth and care. Such a leader, they suggest, is able to infuse political and economic debate with ethical values. In researching trust in schools, Tschannen-Moran and Hoy (2000) make a similar observation. Trust is built when the principal is consistent, competent, fair and honest. Moral actions, even relatively small ones, speak loudly. The authors tell the story of the positive impact on staff of a principal's willingness to apologise for an unfair remark made to a teacher.

The personal element in the building up of the covenant relationship was absolutely central. The covenant, as Vriezen (1970, p.309) notes, was founded on the 'double aspects' of holiness and morality. Vriezen connects these traits with the truth or trustworthiness of God. In Hebrew, the word for truth is connected with a stem meaning 'to steady', 'to hold out'. The Hebrew word for faith is also linked with this: *he'emin* means to look upon God as steadfast, trustworthy. In Yahweh's fidelity and truth 'Yahweh is the reliable God' (Vriezen 1970, p.309). Vriezen concludes his reflections thus:

> We feel…completely justified in maintaining that the ethical element in Yahwism has full justice done to it and that God, the Holy One, is also known in Israel as the morally perfect or rather absolutely Moral God, who will not compromise with anybody in any province of life where justice and truth are at stake. (p.310)

Trust in the covenant from Israel's side was established on the basis of Yahweh's moral character. Trust is not an impersonal commodity. Persons do not identify solely with words and ideas on paper (or on tablets of stone). There needs to be personal influence infusing the values and beliefs formulated into the lives of the organisation's members. The God who is absolutely committed to truth and justice models the exemplary behaviour required of the persons promoting the vision. Obviously those persons are not expected to be perfect. Unless, however, their actions are more orientated to integrity and justice than not, the identification process will struggle.

In this chapter, we have discussed the crucial role of identification in building a strong partnership between management and staff. In seeking to identify the conditions favouring the internalisation of a corporate vision, we turned to both contemporary management theory and covenant theology for inspiration. The long and hard struggle that is covenant experience vividly reinforces the importance organisational theory attaches to both group identity and the reliability and integrity of leaders. For human service organisations (along with all others), the establishment of a strong group identity is challenging. We discussed a clash of visions around the personalist versus instrumentalist question. That there is this dissonance underlines the significance of the open, intelligent and courageous dialogue that we have been advocating.

In the next chapter, trust will again feature. The attention we have been giving to identification will also be carried over. We will analyse partnership and co-operation in the world of business in order to illuminate the situation of the British National Health Service. As has been our pattern, this discussion will be framed by covenant theology.

Notes

1   This is the view, for example, of E. Kutsch. His works have not been translated from the original German. See Nicholson (1986, pp.104–109) for a description of his approach.

2   On the link between social Darwinism and Smithian philosophy, see McCoy (1985, pp.168–169). Adam Smith had a 'providential' view of economic activity. When individuals act self-interestedly in the marketplace there is an 'invisible hand' guiding the process so that at the same time there is a contribution to the common good. Through a link with the social version of Darwinism, the view arose that the law of the survival of the economically fit has a positive social function. Virile businesses contribute most to the commonwealth.

CHAPTER 7

Competition, Co-operation and Trust

From Business to the NHS

In this final chapter, I want to take some concepts and principles from the commercial world and show how they work out in the context of the British National Health Service (the NHS). The relationship between competition and partnership, on the one hand, and the level of trust built into the commercial system, on the other, are central concerns in the business world. Competition, co-operation and system trust or power, then, are the key terms. Interestingly, these also feature in the life of the NHS.

In the world of business, there is a growing recognition of the value of co-operation. That is, more and more enterprises are choosing to make the move from an unstable situation of 'playing the field' of faceless competitors to one in which long-term partnerships are cultivated. Central to the development of a successful partnership is trust. Trust, in turn, is built through the partners committing themselves to a moral contract (Lorenz 1988).

There are two levels at which trust and co-operation in the commercial sphere can be nurtured. There is the level of the system and that of individual enterprises. When there is what some call 'system power' (Lane and Bachmann 1997), a commercial environment conducive to trust is established. A strong and effective group of trade associations, working in conjunction with the legal system, produces binding norms and standards for business. Even when there is a relatively low level of system power, however, it is still possible to develop trust. While the overall business climate may not inspire a high level of confidence, individual firms can take steps which build a strong partnership. They can, for example, show themselves to be reliable, honest and flexible. These actions and attitudes I will call 'partnership investment'.

The dialectic of competition versus co-operation has been at the centre of the political restructuring of the NHS over the last decade. In 1991 the Thatcher government, convinced of the value of competition, introduced an internal market into the NHS in a bid to improve efficiency and quality. Six years later the newly elected, Tony Blair-led New Labour government would make some significant changes. The purchaser–provider split was retained, but the policy rhetoric now centred on co-operation and partnership rather than on competition.

Our pastoral concern in relation to the NHS centres on the level of trust that all parties, especially the patients, have in the Service. Trust in the health system depends, in large part, on the quality of the clinical services provided. Patients want to be assured that the care delivered by health care providers will be first-rate. In the new structure established by the Labour government, 'system power' is expressed through 'clinical governance'. It is a system in which trust boards and the chief executive are held accountable for the quality of the care that is provided.

As in the previous two chapters, I want to use covenant theology to illuminate the discussion. In the covenant, there was both 'system power' and 'partnership investment'. That is to say, there were both institutional and relational elements. I will be suggesting that ultimately the covenant moved on from cult, *Torah* and monarchy (the components of system power) to a very personal 'investment' in the divine–human relationship through the incarnation and the cross/resurrection. As we saw in the last chapter, the ultimate aim of the new covenant is identification with God in Christ through an act of faith. What covenant theology suggests for the NHS (and for business for that matter), I will argue, is that while system power plays an important role in establishing an environment conducive to trust, it is only through relational investment that the goal of identification with a vision is achieved. Put simply, it is not possible to institutionalise moral action and ownership of a vision.

The shape of the chapter is as follows. To begin, I will set the scene for the discussion by describing the realities of competition in the commercial sphere and by indicating that there is a trend to move beyond rivalry to co-operation. As working together requires trust, the second task is to distinguish between personal and system trust. With this discussion as a basis, we will discuss the way in which both 'system power' and 'partnership investment' contribute to the establishment of trust in business. The relationship between these two dynamics will also be analysed in the context of the covenant. I then want to take these various ideas from business and from the covenant and apply them to the case of the NHS. I will attempt to show that the success of clinical governance ultimately depends on the quality of the relationships between the various partners, namely hospital management, clinical staff and patient groups.

From competition to co-operation

There is an interesting dichotomy between the views of economists and those of businesspersons on the role of competition (Moore 1993). In the view of economists, competition is an essential factor in the market system. It has the important role of promoting the utilisation of scarce resources at optimum efficiency. Those engaged in business, on the other hand, see it almost as a 'necessary evil' of the market. Rivalry in business means that the firm is always under pressure and its prosperity under threat. From the perspective of the businessperson, the economic world is loaded with rivals. He or she must contend with customers, suppliers, potential entrants, substitute products and established competitors. The corporate strategist searches for that niche where the firm can get the better of rivals, or at least influence them in its favour. Being in the position of working with a finite market, it is necessary to establish market share to the disadvantage of rivals.

In the new climate of business, however, firms are seeking to co-operate in order to be more competitive. So, for example, in the Silicon Valley in California it is quite common for competitors to work together on research and development projects. In such a specialised and rapidly changing field as computer technology no one firm has within its ranks the knowledge base to advance its products to the desired level. Technical collaboration is a necessity. In other fields of endeavour, firms are opting for short-term alliances to achieve a common goal. They may, for example, wish to produce a sub-assembly, establish a joint venture or enter a new market. Finally, many manufacturing firms are recognising the benefits in establishing a long-term relationship with their suppliers. These working relationships need trust as a lubricant. The establishment of trust in the business world is influenced both by relationships between the agents of the firms and by the activity of national business institutions. That is, trust in the commercial sphere has both a personal and systemic dimension.

Personal and system trust

The German sociologist Niklas Luhmann has produced a most interesting and illuminating analysis of trust in his book *Trust and Power* (hereafter referred to as *TP*). The overarching notion which shapes all of Luhmann's (1979) sociological interpretations is the reduction of complexity. What is fundamental and of prime importance in the functioning of modern societies is the complexity of their social ordering. It is not possible to grasp the realities associated with modern life in their totality. There is, suggests Luhmann, necessarily a process of selection which establishes the way social systems – the economic, the cultural, the political and the religious – will function. That is to say, the systems which structure our social existence do not represent reality as it really is but rather are the consequence of a selection process. The economic, political and cultural systems that we have constructed represent only a segment of the social reality. Choices have been made about which factors and possibilities will be included in social structuring. In a word, the function of social systems is to reduce complexity to a manageable level.

Now Luhmann observes that as well as this complexity in the social sphere there is a complexity in the temporal dimension (*TP*, p.14). It is this temporal complexity which is central in the problem of trust. When a person chooses to trust she involves herself in 'a risky investment' (*TP*, p.24). This is so because she cannot be certain that the future outcome will correspond with her present desires and intentions. There is not just one future possibility but a myriad of possibilities. Thus, the future is not simple; rather, it is complex. This 'problem of time' is bridged by trust. '[T]rust is required for the reduction of a future characterized by more or less indeterminate complexity' (*TP*, p.15). In a sense, the one who trusts is seeking to gain a level of control, to secure a measure of certainty, in the face of the complexity and uncertainty of life-in-relationships.

The way in which we use this 'device' for gaining some control *vis-à-vis* a complex future is socially conditioned. That is, we learn to trust (*TP*, pp.27–28). Our learning begins in the relative safety and security of the family, and then extends to outsiders. Each experience of honesty and reliability strengthens the willingness to trust. Conversely, it may take only one significant betrayal to shatter trust – trust is a fragile commodity.

Luhmann takes his analysis a step further by observing that along with personal trust there is system trust. This 'institutionalised' version of trust is necessary because of social complexity. It is not possible to live life having to establish every encounter, every transaction, on a personal basis. In everyday life we use what Luhmann calls 'communication media' to reduce social complexity. Examples of these 'codes of selection' are money, truth and power. By communication media or codes of selection Luhmann means 'a mechanism additional to language, in other words a code of generalized symbols which guides the transmission of selections' (TP, p.111). So, for example, when we use money we are confident that it actually has power to purchase goods and services. We trust that the monetary system is strong and secure so that when we wake up the next day our financial resources will have much the same worth as the day before. Finally, we have a faith in the monetary system which allows for a delay in the option to buy. That is, we are prepared to save and invest. That this is an example of system trust is evident when one reflects that individuals do not daily contact bank officials and investment brokers in an attempt to establish that the monetary system is secure.

This last observation points to the fact that in modern societies people receive a large array of information in an already simplified form. That is, we rely on others to process facts and figures for us. Thus, *truth* or meaning is another example of a communication medium. When I engage with my doctor, mechanic or solicitor I do not seek to personally verify every statement that is made, every action that is performed. Rather, I trust in a system of accreditation which confirms that he or she has the requisite knowledge and skill to serve my needs satisfactorily.

Luhmann's last example is political power. At the most basic level, the fact that citizens trust in the political process is evidenced by the fact that they remain in the country confident that life will be relatively satisfactory. Further, the system of institutionalised checks and balances engenders a certain level of trust. While many of us do monitor individual politicians and political actions quite closely, the ordinary person lacks both the skill and the time to analyse constitutional documents and political processes in detail. Trust in the political process, like trust in money and meaning, is established at a system rather than at a personal level.

Building trust: System power and partnership investment

In a comparative study of inter-firm relations in Britain and Germany, sociologists Lane and Bachmann (1997) take Luhmann's ideas a step further. They suggest that what they call 'system power' is a notion closely related to system trust. Lane and Bachmann recognise that trust is of central importance and of great value in building the partnership between firms; however, they are also aware that it is a fragile commodity. With this in mind, they ask the question whether there is a functional analogue which is more robust. The authors take their lead in the search from Luhmann's idea that power is a 'medium of communication'. Given the complications and intricacies of the general business environment and the particular inter-firm relations, there needs to be a code or medium which manages and shapes that complexity. Business and legal systems, when they are strong and when they complement each other, the authors suggest, create a fund of shared norms, values and expectations which reduces the alternatives for business practice. That is, a code of business conduct is established and opportunistic behaviour is strongly discouraged. Systems are set in place which create a climate of trust in the conduct of business. These systems are able to produce this ethos because they possess power or authority. 'Strong institutional frameworks reduce the risk of trust, but only because and in so far as they embody power. Thus "system power" can be seen as a precondition of "system trust"' (Lane and Bachmann 1997, p.234).

In their study, Lane and Bachmann come to the conclusion that system power is high in Germany and relatively low in Britain. The British pattern of business associability is characterised as 'a pluralistic and lowly integrated system of business associations, with weak representation at the national level' (Lane and Bachmann 1997, p.234). In Germany, on the other hand, they found 'a very orderly and highly integrated hierarchical system, constituting an effective interlocutor for the national state' (Lane and Bachmann 1997, p.234). A strong and influential network of industry associations such as exists in Germany has the power to shape and control the way business is conducted. It sets the norms and standards which are virtually binding on all firms. These guidelines for the conduct of business are called the General Business Conditions (*Allegemeine Geshäfts-bedingungen*). They function, as Lane and Bachmann (1997, p.239) put it, to establish 'a world in common'. In Britain, there is no organisational umbrella with this authority. The ethics of business is something which individual firms, within limits, decide for themselves.

With reference to the legal system, the authors found that German contract law assigns a much higher value to the principle of good faith than does its British counterpart. Notions of mutual responsibility and consideration of interests have a central place in German contract law. That is not to say, of course, that in Britain there is little appreciation of the importance of ethics in contracts. However, the fact that there is an absence of guiding principles, along with the fact that there is generally stricter adherence to the letter of the contract, means that there is a tendency to favour the stronger party in the arrangement. In England, it tends to be the consumer, the authors note, rather than the weaker business partner who is protected. While English judges are conscious of their responsibility to invalidate unfair contract terms, there are no general requirements of good faith. That is, the system lacks power in the terms we are using. The end result is that the stronger party gains an advantage.

> By leaving more discretion to the business partners to decide on the allocation of risks between them English law places individual autonomy above the consideration of common interests and implicitly gives license to the more powerful party. (Lane and Bachmann 1997, p.246)

It might seem from the picture painted by Lane and Bachmann that Germany has a high-trust and Britain a low-trust business environment. This view of things is somewhat misleading, however. There is no doubt that the presence of strong and influential institutional systems contributes significantly to the establishment of a climate of trust in the business world. But even when system power is relatively low, it is still possible for individual firms to effectively build trust. Economists Burchell and Wilkinson (1997) have carried out another comparative study, but this time including Italy in the research, and have come up with some interesting conclusions. They are well aware of the important role of system trust in Germany. They further found that the respondents to their survey identified what they, the authors, called 'substantive' and 'procedural' elements in trust (Burchell and Wilkinson 1997, p.226). In the former category are trust-building *qualities* displayed by business partners. These include attributes such as honesty, reliability, promise-keeping and fairness. The latter category refers to trust-building *processes*. For example, a supplier will over time establish a reputation for timely supply of quality, cost-effective components. Maintaining close personal contact is another important way to establish trust. The emphasis, the authors found, in the British context is on building the business relationship. So, for example, if there is a minor lapse in the working relationship it is quite likely that it would simply be forgiven. A significant number of firms, also, indicated a preparedness to assist or to adjust plans even though they were not contractually obligated to do so.

It seems clear that both system power and partnership investment make their own distinctive and important contributions to positive business relationships. Organisational theorist Walter Powell refers to the former as an 'embedded' form of trust (Powell 1996). In certain societies, firms find themselves embedded in a web of norms, values and expectations. Powell (1996) also refers to a form of trust that is chosen, namely 'rational or calculative trust' (p.62). In this model, trust is 'a rational outcome of an iterated chain of contacts in which farsighted parties recognize the potential benefits of their continued interaction' (Powell 1996, p.62). He goes on to make the important comment that 'we need to recognize the extent to which trust is neither chosen nor embedded but is instead learned and reinforced, hence a product of ongoing interaction and discussion' (Powell 1996, p.63). I want to extend this insight slightly and suggest that, as important and powerful as system trust is, ultimately it cannot ensure that the partners in a business relationship reach the goal of identification. Strong, cohesive institutional structures work to create a climate of fair and just dealing; the cultivation of the partnership, on the other hand, is something the individual firms must do. The ultimate aim in inter-firm relations is for both parties to own each other's preferences. That is, each party reaches the point where it understands the vision of the other and takes it on as their own. To reach this stage in understanding and co-operation obviously requires a considerable degree of investment in the relationship.

With reference to the British scene, Burchell and Wilkinson (1997) found that a significant number of firms are prepared to be flexible both 'beyond' and 'outside' contracts in the interests of the long-term relationship. Being flexible beyond contract terms involves behaviours such as the following: (a) being ready to exchange business information, (b) honouring informal understandings, and (c) a preparedness to re-negotiate terms at any time. Flexibility outside a contract refers to social or interpersonal commitments. For example, there is a readiness to help out in an emergency. Rather than sticking rigidly to the letter of the contract, there is a willingness for give and take. Finally, this kind of flexibility means that occasional faults will simply be overlooked.

When there is this level of investment in the relationship, partners begin both to understand and to trust each other. It is this ongoing interaction and commitment which moves them in the direction of identification. That this is in fact the case has been demonstrated through research carried out by Tsai and Ghosal (1998). In the building up of social capital between business units Tsai and Ghosal identify three key factors, namely the 'structural', the 'cognitive' and the 'relational'. The structural refers to activities designed to build social bonds. Developing a 'shared paradigm' is the aim of the cognitive dimension. And finally, the relational factor refers to trust and trustworthiness. The authors show how these three factors are interlinked. When there is frequent and close contact (the structural) between the members of the various business units there is an opportunity for the actors to develop an understanding, to learn to interpret and appreciate each other's characteristic attitudes and behaviours, each other's valued aims and goals. Over time, it is possible that the actors will develop together a 'shared paradigm', a common vision (identification). When there is a sense that everyone is committed to a common goal there is a confidence that the temptation to opportunism will be denied. The relational bonds (the bonds of trust) are in this case strong. In sum, consistent positive interaction facilitates understanding, a common vision and trust-building.

At this point it will perhaps be instructive to introduce the experience of both Israel and the church in the covenant relationship with God. The relationship with Israel was strengthened both by system power and partnership investment. I suggest, however, that in the end the decisive factor in the covenant is not the institutional, but rather the relational. This is particularly true of the new covenant. God related intimately to God's people through Christ, calling them to identify with him and with the values of the Reign of God.

System power and relational 'investment' in the covenant

It is evident that the covenant between Yahweh and Israel had an institutional form. The three central institutional elements were *Torah*, the cultus and the monarchy. Yahweh's will and purpose was communicated primarily through *Torah* – law or instruction. While this religious instruction was mainly communicated by a priest (see Jer 18:18), the prophet (see Isa 8:16), the wise man (see Prov 3:1, 4:2) and the king (see Isa 2:3) could also perform this function. A reference to the law books will indicate that the scope of *Torah* was very extensive. We find counsel on matters such as cultic observance, moral attitudes, health, the avoidance of unclean foods, sexual matters, social manners, military service, the care of buildings, the protection of slaves and the conservation of the environment. The fact that righteous conduct in virtually every area of personal and corporate life was clearly laid out indicates the power of *Torah*. Moreover, Israel knew that disobedience in relation to the law carried with it the direst consequences. The covenant was in no way unconditional. If the people were faithful in fulfilling their obligations they could be assured of Yahweh's continued blessings. Failure to live faithfully, on the other hand, would bring down the curses of heaven. There were thus two dimensions to the power of *Torah* in the covenant system. First, the people were left in no doubt as to what was expected of them in terms of religious and moral conduct. And second, if they did fall into waywardness, divine chastisement was sure and severe.

Of course, even though they were very aware of the possibility of chastisement, the people were not always faithful to the demands of *Torah*. In this case, there was a need for atonement. Reconciliation with God had a central place in the cultus (see Exod 30:10; Lev 1:4, 5, 6:24–30, 7:1–10, 16). The other key dimensions in the cultic life of Israel were the glorification of God and maintaining fellowship with God (see Lev 1–6). In fact, the three facets were linked. So although the primary purpose of the burnt offering was the bringing of a gift to glorify God, reference to Leviticus 1:4 indicates that it also served to make atonement.

The third element in the power of the covenant system was the monarchy. The king acted as an agent of the divine will and purpose. That a central concern in the divine economy was the protection of the weak and the marginalised is clear from passages such as Exodus 22:21–24:

> Do not mistreat an alien or oppress him, for you were aliens in Egypt. Do not take advantage of a widow or orphan. If you do and they cry out to me, I will certainly hear their cry. My anger will be aroused, and I will kill you with the sword; your wives will become widows and your children fatherless.

To establish justice and righteousness in the land was a primary responsibility of the king. Protecting the interests of the weak was particularly important. In the 72nd psalm we are presented with the royal ideal:

> Endow the king with your justice, O God, the royal son with your righteousness. He will judge your people in righteousness, your afflicted ones with justice. The mountains will bring prosperity to the people, the hills the fruit of righteousness. He will defend the afflicted among the people and save the children of the needy; he will crush the oppressor. (vv.1–4)

Righteousness and justice were ideals which were promoted through preaching. They were also backed up through the power of the theocratic system. God had established the monarchy and given the king power and authority to rule in the land according to the divine will and purpose.

While there is no doubt that the institutional forms served a useful and important role, the deepest intention in the covenant goes beyond those forms and the power associated with them to identification by the people with the ethical norms for interpersonal life established by Yahweh. The Old Testament presents the main purpose of the covenant as the moulding of the people in the spiritual and moral life that God has ordained. In order to realise this goal, it was necessary for God to relate to, to communicate with, the people in a personal way. The prophets were those persons who identified with the vision of Yahweh and were called to proclaim that vision to the nation. A central element in their message was that right conduct rather than faithful participation in the religious system is what God desires. Nicholson (1986) is exactly right when he says:

So far from being a social institution, the covenant represents the refusal of the prophets and their disciples to encapsulate Yahweh's relationship with his people in institutions, and to insist that it depends on a moral commitment on both sides which needs to be continually reaffirmed in faithful conduct, not taken for granted (as were institutions such as the monarchy in the ancient world) as though it were part of the order of nature. (p.216)

The 8th century BC prophets – Isaiah, Hosea, Amos and Micah – in their various ways were saying to the people of Israel that their way of life could not be reconciled with God's teaching. They had moved a long way from the divine plan for personal and social life in the world. The area of deviation they concentrated on varied. For example, Hosea was primarily concerned with apostasy. The people were 'whoring' after the gods of fertility. Isaiah, Amos and Micah highlighted the sin of injustice against the poor. While there were different grounds for indictment of the people, all four prophets raised time and again the issue of the failures of Israel in the ethical sphere. In particular, they proclaimed the message that what the Lord requires is not a lavish cultus but holy and just conduct (see Isa 1:1–10; Hos 6:6; Amos 4:4–5, 5:21–25; Mic 6:6–8).

The central role of the prophets in the covenant indicates a going beyond institutional forms in order to interact in a personal way with the people. *Torah* established clearly enough the parameters for the life of Israel. The people knew more or less what was expected of them. Of course, there would always be the question of exactly what applying *Torah* meant in the changing circumstances of the nation. But in general, the people were aware of the kind of ethical conduct expected of them. It is one thing to have laid out a system of rules, norms and expectations. Finding the commitment and the will to live faithful to that spiritual and moral code is something else again. What the record of the prophetic tradition demonstrates is that it is only through intense personal contact that people will be moved to identify with a moral vision.

As we saw in the last chapter, this concentrated personal influence was given a radical interpretation by the prophet Jeremiah in announcing the new covenant (Jer 31:31–34). Through a miraculous action God would personally write the law on the hearts and minds of the people. The personal investment in the relationship with God's people reaches an apogee with the coming of the Son. In the imagery of the parable of the tenants (Matt 21:33–46), the first agents charged with the responsibility of inculcating the holy vision in the occupants of the vineyard were the servants (the prophets). The tenants, sadly, turned their hearts and minds away from the proclamation and abused some and killed other messengers. Finally, the landowner decided that he would send his Son, believing that they would surely take notice of him. Not so! He too was killed; but the rejected One nevertheless effected a wonderful reversal and set the seal on the whole project of renewal.

Over time in covenant history the personal investment in the divine–human partnership intensified. *Torah* established quite clearly what the divine expectations were in the spiritual and moral spheres. The various institutional forms gave a very definite shape to the personal and communal life of the people. A climate of moral conduct was created. But when an opportunity to step on others to advance one's own interests presented itself, many could not say 'no'. There was always an urgent need to call people back into line with the covenant vision, and this required a personal engagement. Starting with the prophets, moving to God's direct action in the new covenant, and culminating in the absolutely personal communication in and through the Son, there was a long history of intense dialogue between God and the people aimed at moving them to identify with the divine plan. There is in covenant theology a vivid verification of the notion in the commercial world that while system power has the very important function of creating a business environment conducive to trust, it is only through consistently positive contact that the partners in a commercial venture will develop a 'shared paradigm'. There are limits on what system power can achieve. Interpersonal engagement at a number of levels is necessary if the parties are to reach the point of identification.

What I have been aiming at in discussing at length the roles of system power and partnership investment in both the commercial world and covenantal life is to gather some principles that will illuminate the situation of the NHS. These themes, along with that of competition versus co-operation, are prominent in the ongoing debates over its functioning.

System power and relational strength in the NHS

The debate in the commercial world over the respective merits of competition and co-operation has also occupied the minds of those responsible for the NHS. When Conservative governments were in power in the 1990s a commitment to competition guided government policy. With the coming to power of New Labour, however, an emphasis on collaboration and partnership was promoted. In an attempt to increase the quality of health services, a programme of clinical governance was set in place. This constituted the 'system power' in the new approach. I want now to show that the principle from the covenant applied to business partnerships – that the personal moral commitments of the partners is of fundamental importance – also applies to the NHS.

The Conservative government led by Margaret Thatcher, inspired to a large extent by the ideas of American experts, especially Alain Enthoven, replaced the state bureaucracy of the NHS by an internal market in health care. (For information on the operation of the internal market in the NHS, see Ham and Maynard 1994; Klein 1999; Le Grand 1999; Newman 1995; Royce 1995.) This was not a free market but rather a managed one. The government provided the finances and operated a number of market controls. While there was competition between independent suppliers to provide the service, it was carefully managed (Ham and Maynard 1994; Royce 1995). The fundamental principle of the market economy is that effective operators will be rewarded with a healthy profit and will prosper, while inefficient operators will miss out. Those enterprises whose level of competitiveness is very low will eventually fall by the wayside. In the managed market of the NHS, this principle did not apply. The providers (hospital trusts) were required to operate as non-profit bodies. Further, struggling hospitals were not allowed to fall over. To avoid the socially and politically undesirable event of a hospital closure, the government came to the rescue.

The quasi-market in secondary health care involved a separation of 'purchasers' from 'providers' of health services. As was the case with the old bureaucratic system, purchasers were funded from tax revenue. Providers operated in a semi-independent fashion, managing their own budgets and financing them from contracts with purchasers. It was at this point that the element of competition was introduced. Hospitals and other secondary care suppliers were required to compete for contracts.

There were two kinds of purchasers. On the one hand, there were district health authorities which were allocated a budget to purchase secondary care based on the size and the other demographic features of the district's population. On the other hand, there was the general practice (GP) fundholder. A GP practice needed to have a certain-sized patient list in order to qualify as a fundholder. A GP fundholder was given a budget to purchase a more limited range of secondary treatments on behalf of its patients (usually elective surgery).

In relation to service provision, hospitals and the providers of other services became independent 'trusts'. They contracted with health authorities and GP fundholders to provide services. In operating their 'business', they could make their own decisions in relation to pay, skill-mix and service delivery. However, there were also certain constraints on their operations. As we have already noted, they were bound by central directives concerning pricing and investment, and they were not allowed to retain any surpluses they generated.

So much for the philosophy and operation of the internal market under the Conservatives. But how well did it fare? While there is relatively little empirical evidence available, the general consensus seems to be that it performed neither as well as its supporters had hoped, nor as disastrously as its critics had predicted (Klein 1999; Le Grand 1999; Smith 2002). What is interesting is that it may well have been that a fundamental reason for the low impact of the internal market was that the primary motivation of the health care agents was the building of trust rather than the promotion of competition (Le Grand 1999). For markets to operate effectively, individuals need to act aggressively to knock over the competition. They need to be single-minded in promoting their own interests. Le Grand (1999) observes, however, that those working in the NHS – doctors, nurses, managers and ancillary staff – did not want to operate in this manner. Up until this point, their work was characterised by trusting relationships, professional discretion and long-standing co-operation. It was this style of operation rather than the aggressive approach of the market that tended to prevail. Further evidence that without the internalisation of a vision a programme will falter.

In any case, the internal market was not to last – at least not in the form just described. While the separation of purchasers from providers was to continue under New Labour, a shift from competition to co-operation was promoted. In the mid-1990s, Labour's spokespersons used the language of partnership (Delamothe 1995). They suggested that the idea of social partnership so central to enlightened industrial relations should be translated to the NHS as health partnership. The vision consisted of the various health partners – health care professionals, health authorities, managers, accountants, patients – all working in concert in a patient-centred ethos.

Recent events indicate that the commitment to such a vision is wavering. There have been moves, especially from Prime Minister Tony Blair, to give more emphasis to the market and to competition (Dean 2003a, 2003b; Dixon 2002). At the forefront of this move is the proposal for the introduction of foundation hospitals (Dean 2002, 2003a; Dixon 2002). These hospitals will be given considerable scope in shaping their operations. Hospital management will be free to do the following: pay extra supplements to staff and change terms and conditions of work; use funds generated through land sales; retain surpluses; and raise capital for new developments through private financial channels. According to the Labour government, this injection of a new competitive element into the health care system will be complemented by a resurrection of the old co-operative or mutual society (Dean 2003a). The election of a majority of the hospital's governing body is to be the responsibility of local people, patients and staff, and a lock on assets will stop them from being demutualised. Foundation hospitals would continue to belong to the people, but they would also be given certain operating freedoms associated with private enterprise.

Clearly the way governments in Britain have approached the co-operation/competition mix in health care is a tale with a number of twists and turns in it. The quality in the system has been connected to a greater or lesser extent with competitive operation. Certainly the Conservative government of the early 1990s saw competition between providers as central in enhancing the quality of health services. When New Labour introduced its changes, however, clinical governance occupied centre stage. This is not to imply that in the old approach there were no formal quality guidelines in place. Clinical governance develops existing systems such as clinical audit, quality assurance, risk management and continuous professional development. What is new is a blueprint for combining these elements in a synergistic way (Pilgrim 1999). Clinical governance can be succinctly defined as a statutory duty for ongoing improvement of the quality of patient care. However, Dale, Croft and Kenyon (1999) point out that the definition in the government's 1997 white paper, entitled 'The New NHS – Modern, Dependable', is much broader than this. There it is described as:

> A new initiative...to assure and improve clinical standards at local level throughout the NHS. This includes action to ensure that risks are avoided, adverse events are rapidly detected...good practice is rapidly disseminated and systems are in place to ensure continuous improvements in clinical care. (cited in Dale *et al.* 1999, p.22)

It is a system, then, with four main components: improving clinical effectiveness, professional development, continuous quality improvement, and risk management (Dale *et al.* 1999; Scally and Donaldson 1998). The health care management has a statutory duty of care in relation to these areas. Clinical governance dictates that trust boards and the chief executive are accountable for the quality of the care that is provided. In the language we have used in relation to the commercial world, it is aimed at strengthening system power. The aim is to build up the level of trust in the health care system.

Here I believe that both intelligent commercial practice and covenantal theology can make an important contribution. In the end, the tools of system power depend on the moral quality of the relationships shared by the various agents. Enlightened business leaders are increasingly talking about the value in a moral contract. Successful co-operation requires personal investment from all those involved. They recognise that consistent positive behaviour builds the trust that is the foundation for a flourishing commercial partnership. Despite the very different context, the Hebrew Scriptures speak a similar language. Time and again the covenant system was fractured through the frailties of the people. God communicated personally through the prophets and, most decisively, through Jesus in order to renew and to transform the vision. It was the quality of the relationship between God and the people that made the covenant a living reality.

Those who comment on clinical governance make a point that reflects these principles. Scally and Donaldson (1998) argue that the quality of the working relationship between senior managers and health professionals is at the heart of clinical governance. Halligan and Donaldson (2001) share this view. They contend that what is needed is for hospital leadership to communicate 'the vision, values, and methods' of clinical governance to staff in such a way that they are internalised. When this happens, everyone works together with 'a common and consistent purpose'.

The covenant experience reminds us that the consistent communication of Yahweh's values and purposes was backed by Yahweh's moral commitment to the people. Halligan and Donaldson (2001) suggest that along with the support of professional development, there is another equally important function for the hospital leadership in relation to clinical governance. It must ensure that staff feel valued, are included in ideas generation and policy decisions, and that staff problems and concerns are heard and acted upon. In a word, clinical governance is ultimately only as good as the quality of the professional relationships in the hospital.

It is easy when talking about the quality of health care to focus exclusively on the roles of management and clinical staff. Importantly, Winter (1999) contends that the patient group must also be seen as a partner in clinical governance:

> Whilst Quality and Clinical Effectiveness might be seen as being within the domain of the clinician and health professional, the full potential to improve the quality of the service will only be achieved if there is real and meaningful participation of patients and users of the service. (p.28)

Of vital importance here, Winter points out, is an effective complaints and comment system.

Clinical governance has the potential to build the level of trust in the health care system. Ultimately, though, its effectiveness depends on the quality of the working relationship between the three main partners, namely management, clinical staff and patient groups.

What I have been arguing in this final chapter is that in relation to the health care sphere both intelligent business practice and covenant theology can make an important contribution. Both system power and personal investment are important. In the end, it is the quality of personal relationships between the partners that makes the system effective. A covenant ultimately depends on the moral capacity of the partners. The vision needs to be internalised. In health care, institutionalised quality monitoring will only be optimally effective in the context of a strong working relationship between the partners. It is their commitment to each other and to the shared vision that makes the system work.

Conclusion

In this book, I have attempted a theological and ethical analysis of relationships in human service provision. My concern has been a pastoral one. The aim has been to identify those attitudes, behaviours and personal capacities which humanise or spiritualise a series of working relationships. An attempt has been made to describe the factors in the way various human services are delivered, on the one hand, and in the organisational life supporting those services, on the other, which contribute to the psychological and spiritual well-being of the various actors.

In the first half of the book, I developed the notion that self-communication is a virtue in the personal service professions. While technical competencies play an important role in personal service, the impact of factors such as empathy, warmth, compassion, respect, support and affirmation needs to be fully appreciated. Moreover, charm, that quality which is an expression of the unity of *agape* and *eros,* is not given nearly enough attention in the literature. Because it has the capacity to refresh the spirit and reveal the self to itself, it is a powerful asset for those engaged in personal service. It may not be going too far to suggest that these relational capacities are at the very heart of vocations such as nursing, midwifery, teaching and counselling. While, to be sure, a personal service practitioner must be skilled, if she lacks the virtue of self-communication she cannot be true to her calling. The most important part of what it means to be nurse, a teacher or a counsellor is missing.

The idea of partnerships in organisational life occupied us in the second half of the book. I wanted to show that the covenant offers a model of genuine partnership. God engaged in an intense personal dialogue with Israel, and later with the church, aimed at bringing the people to a point of internalisation of the divine project for them and for the world. Along the way, God always acted loyally and faithfully. The promotion of the well-being of the people and, beyond them, of the world was at all times the driving aim.

For those who recognise that humanising life in an organisation contributes substantially to its effectiveness, the theology of the covenant provides a very useful resource. Creating an environment where staff members feel they are recognised and valued, where they are given opportunities for creative self-expression and where, in a word, they feel they truly belong involves a significant investment in time and resources. It is an investment, however, that effective managers know is vitally important.

A key factor in the life of a vital, energetic and harmoniously functioning partnership is trust. In the dialogue between God and God's people, trust was built on God's capacity for inclusion in their world and for a faithful response to the concerns and hopes they expressed. It is God's engagement in and through the covenant which provides the model for the dialogue between management and staff. The goal of the covenant was always to bring the people to a point of full identification with God's plan. Within an organisation, the process of identification begins with inclusion and committed action. It is when both parties show a readiness to actively reach into the other's concerns, fears, hopes and aspirations and, beyond that, to respond with energy, commitment and integrity that trust is built. When the level of personal investment is high, it will be a trust grounded in identification. When there is an internalisation of each other's preferences, a partnership in the fullest sense is established, and the benefits, both for individuals and for the organisation, are considerable. In human service organisations (along with all others), however, the establishment of a cohesive sense of identity is often problematic. In general, the clash of visions we discussed revolves around the personalist versus instrumentalist question. To be more specific, we looked at dissonance in relation to the care/cure balance, humanised versus medicalised birth and justice versus elitism. That there are these clashes is clearly a matter of some concern. Both individuals and organisations are suffering. The principles that we developed for an intelligent, open and courageous dialogue are vitally important if there is to be any significant movement towards a common vision.

Trusting relationships between organisations are built around 'system power' and 'partnership investment'. In the covenant, both these realities were present. That is to say, there were both institutional and relational elements. We have seen that ultimately the covenant moved on from cult, *Torah* and monarchy (the components of system power) to a very personal 'investment' in the divine–human relationship through the incarnation and the cross/resurrection. The ultimate aim of the new covenant is identification with God in Christ through an act of faith.

Drawing on the experience of both enlightened business and covenant life, I made the point that it is the quality of the personal relationships between the partners that makes the system effective. A covenant ultimately depends on the moral capacity of the partners. The vision needs to be internalised. Applying this principle to health care, I argued that institutionalised quality monitoring will only be optimally effective when there are strong working relationships between the partners. And here I identified three partners, namely management, clinical staff and patient groups. It is their commitment to each other and to the shared vision that will make the system work.

The relationships associated with human service provision – as in all other forms of work – are too often characterised by alienation, mistrust, infidelity, egoism and stress. Attending to the three key ideals of self-communication, belonging and trust, I have attempted to shape a normative vision for working relationships in the personal service area. If these relationships are to take on an increasingly truly human or spiritual character, the actors will need to intensify their commitment to these ideals.

References

Adams, R. (1987) *The Virtue of Faith and Other Essays in Philosophical Theology*. Oxford: Oxford University Press.

Andolsen, B.H. (1988) 'The social self at the VDT: Exploring the advantages and limitations of the relational model of agency.' In D. Yeager (ed) *Annual of the Society of Christian Ethics*. Washington, DC: Georgetown University Press.

Aquinas, T. (1969) *Summa Theologiae*, Blackfriars edition. London: Eyrie and Spottiswoode.

Aquinas, T. (1988a) 'Commentary on Nichomachean Ethics.' In M. Clark (ed) *An Aquinas Reader*. New York: Fordham University Press.

Aquinas, T. (1988b) 'On truth.' In M. Clark (ed) *An Aquinas Reader*. New York: Fordham University Press.

Aquinas (1988c) 'Debated questions.' In M. Clark (ed) *An Aquinas Reader*. New York: Fordham University Press.

Aristotle (1984) *Nichomachean Ethics*. In J. Barnes (ed) *The Complete Works of Aristotle*, Revised Oxford Translation, Vol. 2. Princeton: Princeton University Press.

Augustine (1991) *Confessions*, trans. by H. Chadwick. Oxford: Oxford University Press.

Avis, P. (1989) *Eros and the Sacred*. London: SPCK.

Bentham, J. (1970) [1789] *An Introduction to the Principles of Morals and Legislation*. London: Athlone Press.

Bradshaw, A. (1999) 'The virtue of nursing: The covenant of care.' *Journal of Medical Ethics 25*, 6, 477–481.

Bright, J. (1979) *Covenant and Promise*. London: SCM Press.

Brophy, J. (1986) 'Teacher influences on student achievement.' *American Psychologist 41*, 10, 1069–1076.

Browning, D. (1976) *The Moral Context of Pastoral Care*. Philadelphia: Westminster Press.

Browning, D. (1987) *Religious Thought and the Modern Psychologies*. Philadelphia: Fortress Press.

Browning, D. (1992) 'Altruism and Christian love.' *Zygon 27*, 4, 421–436.

Brownsberger, M.L. (1995) 'Christian faith and business: A story.' In M. Stackhouse, D.P. McCann, S.J. Roels and P.N. Williams (eds) *On Moral Business: Classical and Contemporary Resources for Ethics in Economic Life*. Grand Rapids: Eerdmans.

Brueggemann, W. (1979) 'Covenanting as human vocation.' *Interpretation 33*, 115–129.

Brueggemann, W. (1997) *Theology of the Hebrew Scriptures: Testimony, Dispute, Advocacy*. Minneapolis: Fortress Press.

Brueggemann, W. (1999) *The Covenanted Self: Explorations in Law and Covenant*. Minneapolis: Fortress Press.

Bruner, J. (1996) *The Culture of Education*. Cambridge, MA: Harvard University Press.

Buber, M. (1947) *Between Man and Man*, trans. by R. Gregor Smith. London: Routledge and Kegan Paul.

Buber, M. (1957) 'Elements of the interhuman.' *Psychiatry 20*, 105–113.

Buber, M. (1990) *A Believing Humanism*. London: Humanities Press International. First published in 1967.

Bugental, J.F.T. (1987) *The Art of the Psychotherapist*. New York: Norton.

Burchell, B. and Wilkinson, F. (1997) 'Trust, business relationships and the contractual environment.' *Cambridge Journal of Economics 21*, 217–237.

Campbell, A. (1984) *Moderated Love: A Theology of Professional Care.* London: SPCK.

Castel, R. (1996) 'Work and usefulness to the world.' *International Labour Review 135*, 6, 615–622.

Caudron, S. (1997) 'The search for meaning at work.' *Training and Development 51*, 9, 24–27.

Clements, R.E. (1978) *Hebrew Scriptures Theology: A Fresh Approach.* London: Marshall, Morgan and Scott.

Cooper, P. and McIntyre, D. (1996) 'The importance of power-sharing in classroom learning.' In M. Hughes (ed) *Teaching and Learning in Changing Times.* Oxford: Blackwell Publishers.

Creed, W.E.D. and Miles, R. (1996) 'Trust in organizations: A conceptual framework linking organizational forms, managerial philosophies, and the opportunity costs of controls.' In R. Kramer and T. Tyler (eds) *Trust in Organizations: Frontiers of Theory and Research.* Thousand Oaks, CA: Sage Publications.

Dale, R., Croft, A. and Kenyon, M. (1999) 'Implementing clinical governance.' *Healthcare Quality 4*, 3, 22–25.

Dean, M. (2002) 'Government gives hospitals greater independence.' *The Lancet 359*, 9321, 1928.

Dean, M. (2003a) 'UK government reveals plans to give hospitals more control.' *The Lancet 361*, 9363, 1110ff.

Dean, M. (2003b) 'Labour presses on with health service reforms.' *The Lancet 361*, 9373, 1960–1961.

Delamothe, T. (1995) 'Margaret Beckett's third way: Cooperation and partnership.' *British Medical Journal 311*, 6996, 13ff.

Dinham, S. and Scott, C. (1996) *The Teacher 2000 Project: A Study of Teacher Satisfaction, Motivation and Health.* Nepean: University of Western Sydney.

Dixon, J. (2002) 'Foundation hospitals.' *The Lancet 360*, 9349, 1900–1901.

Dodd, A.W. (2001) 'From survival to self-actualization: Reflections on teaching and teacher education.' *The High School Journal 84*, 3, 13–18.

Eakin, J. and MacEachen, E. (1998) 'Health and the social relations of work: A study of the health-related experiences of employees in small workplaces.' *Sociology of Health and Illness 20*, 6, 896–914.

Evans, D. (1980) *Struggle and Fulfilment.* London: Collins.

Flint, C. (1995) *Communicating Midwifery: Twenty Years of Experience.* Hale, Cheshire: Books for Midwives Press.

Frankena, W. (1963) *Ethics.* Englewood Cliffs, NJ: Prentice-Hall.

Friedman, M. (1985) *The Healing Dialogue in Psychotherapy.* New York: Jason Aronson.

Friedman, M. (1992) *Dialogue and the Human Image: Beyond Humanistic Psychology.* London: Sage.

Friedman, M. (1998) 'Buber's philosophy as the basis for dialogical psychotherapy and contextual therapy.' *Journal of Humanistic Psychology 38*, 1, 25–40.

Fukuyama, F. (1992) *The End of History and the Last Man.* London: Penguin Books.

Fukuyama, F. (1995) *Trust: The Social Virtues and the Creation of Prosperity.* London: Hamish Hamilton.

Gastmans, C. (1998) 'Interpersonal relations in nursing: A philosophical-ethical analysis of the work of Hildegard E. Peplau.' *Journal of Advanced Nursing 28*, 6, 1312–1319.

Gerkin, C. (1986) *Widening the Horizons: Pastoral Responses to a Fragmented Society.* Philadelphia: Westminster Press.

Gerkin, C. (1991) *Prophetic Pastoral Practice: A Christian Vision of Life Together.* Nashville: Abingdon Press.

Gibbs, R. (1989) 'Substitution: Marcel and Levinas.' *Philosophy and Theology 4*, 171–185.

Graham, E. (1996) *Transforming Practice: Pastoral Theology in an Age of Uncertainty*. London: Mowbray.

Green, J., Coupland, V. and Kitzinger, J. (1990) 'Expectations, experiences, and psychological outcomes of childbirth: A prospective study of 825 women.' *Birth 17*, 1, 15–23.

Halligan, A. and Donaldson, L. (2001) 'Implementing clinical governance: Turning vision into reality.' *British Medical Journal 322*, 7299, 1413–1417.

Ham, C. and Maynard, A. (1994) 'Managing the NHS market.' *British Medical Journal 308*, 6932, 845ff.

Hanson, P. (1986) *The People Called: The Growth of Community in the Bible*. San Francisco: Harper and Row.

Hartrick, G. (1997) 'Relational capacity: The foundation for interpersonal nursing practice.' *Journal of Advanced Nursing 26*, 3, 523–528.

Hauerwas, S. (1975) *Character and the Christian Life: A Study in Theological Ethics*. San Antonio: Trinity University Press.

Hauerwas, S. (1981) *Vision and Virtue*. Notre Dame: University of Notre Dame Press.

Herman, R. and Gioia, J. (1998) 'Making work meaningful: Secrets of the future-focused corporation.' *Futurist 32*, 9, 24ff.

Herman, S. (1995) 'The potential of building covenants in business corporations.' In M. Stackhouse and D. McCann (eds) *On Moral Business: Classical and Contemporary Sources for Ethics in Economic Life*. Grand Rapids: Eerdmans.

Herman, S. (1997) *Durable Goods: A Covenantal Ethic for Management and Employees*. Notre Dame: University of Notre Dame Press.

Hobson, R. (1985) *Forms of Feeling: The Heart of Psychotherapy*. London: Tavistock Publications.

Hycner, R. (1991) *Between Person and Person: Toward a Dialogical Psychotherapy*. Highland, NY: The Gestalt Journal.

Janssens, L. (1977) 'Norms and priorities in a love ethics.' *Louvain Studies 6*, 207–238.

Kainz, H. (1988) *Ethics in Context*. London: The Macmillan Press.

Kant, I. (1949) [1788] *Fundamental Principles of the Metaphysics of Morals*, trans. by T. Abbott. New York: Bobbs-Merrill.

Kent, B. (1994) 'Moral provincialism.' *Religious Studies 30*, 269–285.

Kitson, A. (2001) 'Nursing leadership: Bringing caring back into the future.' *Quality in Health Care 10*, 1179–1185.

Kitzinger, S. (1988) 'Why women need midwives.' In S. Kitzinger (ed) *The Midwife Challenge*. London: Pandora Press.

Klein, R. (1999) 'Markets, politicians, and the NHS.' *British Medical Journal 319*, 1383–1384.

Kohut, H. (1971) *The Analysis of the Self*. New York: International Universities Press.

Kohut, H. (1977) *The Restoration of the Self*. New York: International Universities Press.

Kohut, H. (1984) *How Does Analysis Cure?* Chicago: University of Chicago.

Kotter, J. and Heskett, J. (1992) *Corporate Culture and Performance*. New York: The Free Press.

Krajewski, R. (1996) 'Enculturating the school: The principal's principles.' *National Association of Secondary School Principals Bulletin 80*, 576, 3ff.

Kramer, R. and Brewer, M. (1984) 'Effects of group identity on resource use in a simulated commons dilemma.' *Journal of Personality and Social Psychology 46*, 5, 1044–1057.

Lane, C. and Bachmann, R. (1997) 'Co-operation in inter-firm relations in Britain and Germany: The role of social institutions.' *British Journal of Sociology 48*, 2, 226–254.

Lantz, J. (1994a) 'Mystery in family therapy.' *Contemporary Family Therapy 16*, 1, 53–66.

Lantz, J. (1994b) 'Marcel's "availability" in existential psychotherapy with couples and families.' *Contemporary Family Therapy 16*, 6, 489–501.

Le Grand, J. (1999) 'Competition, cooperation, or control? Tales from the British National Health Service.' *Health Affairs 18*, 3, 27–39.

Lewicki, R. and Bunker, B.B. (1996) 'Developing and maintaining trust in work relationships.' In R. Kramer and T. Tyler (eds) *Trust in Organizations: Frontiers of Theory and Research*. Thousand Oaks, CA: Sage Publications.

Lorenz, E. (1988) 'Neither friends nor strangers: Informal networks of subcontracting in French industry.' In D. Gambetta (ed) *Trust: Making and Breaking Cooperative Relations*. London: Basil Blackwell.

Luhmann, N. (1979) *Trust and Power*. Chichester: John Wiley and Sons.

Lungren, I. and Dahlberg, K. (1998) 'Women's experience of pain during childbirth.' *Midwifery 14*, 105–110.

MacIntyre, A. (1985) *After Virtue: A Study in Moral Theory*, 2nd edition. London: Duckworth Press.

Mander, A. (1997) 'Teachers' work: Some complex interactions between teachers and their schools.' *Asia-Pacific Journal of Teacher Education 25*, 3, 281–293.

Marcel, G. (1950) *The Mystery of Being*, Vol. I. London: The Harvill Press.

Marcel, G. (1952) *Metaphysical Journal*. London: Rockliff.

Marcel, G. (1964a) 'Phenomenological notes on being in a situation.' In his *Creative Fidelity*. New York: The Noonday Press.

Marcel, G. (1964b) 'Belonging and disposability.' In his *Creative Fidelity*. New York: The Noonday Press.

May, R. (1983) *The Discovery of Being*. New York: W.W. Norton.

McCarthy, M. (1992) 'Empathy: A bridge between.' *The Journal of Pastoral Care 46*, 2, 119–128.

McClendon, J. (1986) *Systematic Theology: Ethics*. Nashville: Abingdon Press.

McComiskey, T. (1985) *The Covenants of Promise: A Theology of the Hebrew Scriptures Covenants*. London: Intervarsity Press.

McCoy, C. (1985) *Management of Values: The Ethical Difference in Corporate Policy and Performance*. Boston: Pitman Publishing.

McFadyen, A. (1990) *The Call to Personhood: A Christian Theory of the Individual in Social Relationships*. Cambridge: Cambridge University Press.

McInerny, R. (1993) 'Ethics.' In N. Kretzmann and E. Stump (eds) *The Cambridge Companion to Aquinas*. Cambridge: Cambridge University Press.

McKay, S. (1998) 'The route to true autonomous practice for midwives.' *MIDIRS Midwifery Digest 8*, 1, 17–18.

Méda, D. (1996) 'New perspectives on work as value.' *International Labour Review 135*, 6, 633–643.

Meilaender, G. (1984) *The Theory and Practice of Virtue*. Notre Dame: University of Notre Dame Press.

Mendenhall, G. and Herion, G. (1992) 'Covenant.' In D. Freedman (ed) *The Anchor Bible Dictionary*, Vol. 1. New York: Doubleday.

Moore, G. (1993) 'Beyond competition.' In J. Davies (ed) *God and the Marketplace: Essays on the Morality of Wealth Creation*. London: IEA Health and Welfare Unit.

Morgan, G. (1986) *Images of Organization*. Beverley Hills: Sage Publications.

Most, W. (1967) 'A biblical theology of redemption in a covenant framework.' *Catholic Biblical Quarterly 29*, 1–19.

Mückenberger, U. (1996) 'Towards a new definition of the employment relationship.' *International Labour Review 135*, 6, 683–695.

Newman, P. (1995) 'Interview with Alain Enthoven: Is there convergence between Britain and the United States in the organisation of health services?' *British Medical Journal 310*, 6995, 1652ff.

Nicholson, E. (1986) *God and His People: Covenant and Theology in the Old Testament.* Oxford: Clarendon Press.

Nouwen, H. (1972) *The Wounded Healer.* New York: Doubleday.

Nouwen, H. (1996) *Can You Drink the Cup?* Notre Dame: Ave Maria Press.

Nygren, A. (1932) *Agape and Eros,* Pt. I. London: SPCK.

Nygren, A. (1939) *Agape and Eros,* Pt. II, Vol. II. London: SPCK.

O'Connor, M. (2002) '"Good girls" or autonomous professionals?' *MIDIRS Midwifery Digest 12,* 2, 159–164.

Odent, M. (1996) 'Knitting needles, cameras, and electronic fetal monitors.' *MIDIRS Midwifery Digest 6,* 3, 304–306.

Outka, G. (1972) *Agape: An Ethical Analysis.* New Haven: Yale University Press.

Outka, G. (1992) 'Universal love and impartiality.' In E. Santuri and W. Werpehowski (eds) *The Love Commandments: Essays in Christian Ethics and Moral Philosophy.* Washington, DC: Georgetown University Press.

Pattison, S. (1994) *Pastoral Care and Liberation Theology.* Cambridge: Cambridge University Press.

Pembroke, N. (2002) *The Art of Listening: Dialogue, Shame and Pastoral Care.* Grand Rapids: Eerdmans; Edinburgh: T and T Clark.

Pilgrim, D. (1999) 'Making the best of clinical governance.' *Journal of Mental Health 8,* 1, 1–2.

Plato (1997) 'The symposium.' In J. Cooper (ed) *Plato: Complete Works.* Cambridge: Hackett Publishing.

Poling, J. (1988) 'An ethical framework for pastoral care.' *The Journal of Pastoral Care 42,* 4, 299–306.

Poling, J. (1996) *Deliver us from Evil: Resisting Racial and Gender Oppression.* Minneapolis: Fortress Press.

Porter, J. (1990) *The Recovery of Virtue: The Relevance of Aquinas for Christian Ethics.* Louiseville: Westminister/John Knox Press.

Powell, W. (1996) 'Trust-based forms of governance.' In R. Kramer and T. Tyler (eds) *Trust in Organizations: Frontiers of Theory and Research.* Thousand Oaks, CA: Sage Publications.

Preuss, H.D. (1996) *Hebrew Scriptures Theology,* Vol. II. Edinburgh: T and T Clark.

Quinn, D. and Jones, T. (1995) 'An agent morality view of business policy.' *Academy of Management Review 20,* 1, 22–42.

Rahner, K. (1961) 'Concerning the relationship between nature and grace: The supernatural existential.' In his *Theological Investigations,* Vol. I. London: Darton, Longman and Todd.

Rahner, K. (1969) 'Anonymous Christians.' In his *Theological Investigations,* Vol. VI. London: Darton, Longman and Todd.

Ray, M. and Turkel, M. (2002) 'The transformative process for nursing in workplace redevelopment.' *Nursing Administrative Quarterly 26,* 2, 1–14.

Repetti, R. (1987) 'Individual and common components of the social environment at work and psychological well-being.' *Journal of Personality and Social Psychology 52,* 4, 710–720.

Repetti, R. and Cosmos, K. (1991) 'The quality of the social environment at work and job satisfaction.' *Journal of Applied Social Psychology 21,* 10, 840–854.

Robinson, J. (1997) 'Can we measure empathy?' *British Journal of Midwifery 5,* 1, 44–45.

Roeser, R., Midgley, C. and Urdan, T. (1996) 'Perceptions of the school psychological environment and early adolescents' psychological and behavioral functioning in the school: The mediating role of goals and belonging.' *Journal of Educational Psychology 88,* 3, 408–422.

Rogers, C. (1969) *Freedom to Learn.* Columbus, OH: Charles E. Merrill Publishing Company.

Rogers, C. (1980) *A Way of Being.* Boston: Houghton Mifflin Co.

Rogers, C. (1990a) [1958] 'The characteristics of a helping relationship.' In H. Kirschenbaum and V. Land Henderson (eds) *The Carl Rogers Reader.* London: Constable.

Rogers, C. (1990b) [1986] 'A client-centered/person-centered approach to therapy.' In H. Kirschenbaum and V. Land Henderson (eds) *The Carl Rogers Reader*. London: Constable.

Ross, C. (1992) 'Education, control at work, and job satisfaction.' *Social Science Research 21*, 134–148.

Royce, R. (1995) 'Observations on the NHS internal market: Will the dodo have the last laugh?' *British Medical Journal 311*, 7002, 431ff.

Scally, G. and Donaldson, L. (1998) 'Clinical governance and the drive for quality improvement in the new NHS in England.' *British Medical Journal 317*, 4, 61–65.

Schneider, B. (1987) 'The people make the place.' *Personnel Psychology 40*, 437–453.

Shapiro, D., Sheppard, B. and Cheraskin, L. (1992) 'Business on a handshake.' *Negotiation Journal 8*, 4, 365–377.

Sheldrake, P. (1994) *Befriending Our Desires*. London: Darton, Longman and Todd.

Shepphard, B. and Tuchinsky, M. (1996) 'Micro-OB and the network organization.' In R. Kramer and T. Tyler (eds) *Trust in Organizations: Frontiers of Theory and Research*. Thousand Oaks, CA: Sage Publications.

Siddiqui, J. (1999) 'The therapeutic relationship in midwifery.' *British Journal of Midwifery 7*, 2, 111–114.

Skinner, E. and Belmont, M. (1993) 'Motivation in the classroom: Reciprocal effects of teacher behavior and student engagement across the school year.' *Journal of Educational Psychology 85*, 4, 571–581.

Slote, M. (1992) *From Morality to Virtue*. Oxford: Oxford University Press.

Smith, P. (2002) 'Performance management in British health care: Will it deliver?' *Health Affairs 21*, 3, 103ff.

Stolorow, R., Brandchaft, D. and Atwood, G.E. (1987) *Psychoanalytic Treatment: An Intersubjective Approach*. Hillsdale, NJ: The Analytic Press.

Strachan, J. (1999) 'Feminist educational leadership: Locating the concepts in practice.' *Gender and Education 11*, 3, 309–322.

Tolbert, P. and Moen, P. (1998) 'Men's and women's definitions of good jobs: Similarities and differences by age across time.' *Work and Occupation 25*, 2, 168–194.

Tsai, W. and Ghosal, S. (1998) 'Social capital and value creation: The role of intrafirm networks.' *Academy of Management Journal 41*, 4, 464–476.

Tschannen-Moran, M. and Hoy, W. (2000) 'A multidisciplinary analysis of the nature, meaning, and measurement of trust.' *Review of Educational Research 70*, 4, 547–593.

van den Berg, R. (2002) 'Teachers' meanings regarding educational practice.' *Review of Educational Research 72*, 4, 577–625.

von Rad, G. (1975) *Old Testament Theology*, Vol. I. London: SCM Press.

Vriezen, Th. (1970) *An Outline of Old Testament Theology*. London: Basil Blackwell.

Wagner, M. (1998) 'Autonomy: The central issue of midwifery.' *MIDIRS Midwifery Digest 8*, 1, 19–21.

Wagner, M. (2002) 'Fish can't see water: The need to humanize birth.' *MIDIRS Midwifery Digest 12*, 2, 213–220.

Walton, J. (1994) *Covenant: God's Purpose, God's Plan*. Grand Rapids: Zondervan Publishing House.

Winstead, B., Derlega, V., Montgomery, M. and Pilkington, C. (1995) 'The quality of friendships at work and job satisfaction.' *Journal of Social and Personal Relationships 12*, 2, 199–215.

Winter, M. (1999) 'Clinical governance – Getting beyond a new management mantra?' *Healthcare Quality 4*, 3, 26–29.

Wolf, S. (1982) 'Moral saints.' *The Journal of Philosophy 79*, 8, 419–439.

Yalom, I. (1980) *Existential Psychotherapy*. New York: Basic Books.

Subject Index

Name Index

Adams, R. 85
Andolsen, B.H. 116–117
Aquinas, T. 34–35, 43–47, 48, 51–52, 72–73
Aristotle 34, 37, 39–43, 47–48
Atwood, G.E. 70
Augustine 87–88
Avis, P. 86

Bachmann, R. 154–155
Belmont, M. 60, 63
Bentham, J. 35–36
Blair, T. 150, 164
Bradshaw, A. 116
Brandchaft, D. 70
Brewer, M. 144
Bright, J. 104, 106, 128
Brophy, J. 62
Browning, D. 9–10, 29
Brownsberger, M.L. 124
Brueggemann, W. 98–100, 103–105, 117
Bruner, J. 60–63, 65–66
Buber, M. 16, 19–23, 55, 68, 71, 80, 91, 98, 100, 114, 136
Bugental, J. 67–68
Bunker, B.B. 142, 143
Burchell, B. 155–156

Campbell, A. 11, 54
Castel, R. 110–111
Candron, S. 119
Chernskin, L. 108, 141–2
Cicero 35
Clements, R. 106–107
Cooper, P. 64
Cosmos, K. 113
Coupland, V. 56
Creed, W.D. 133
Croft, A. 165

Dahlberg, K. 58
Dale, R. 165
Dean, M. 164
Delamothe, 164
Dinham, S. 112
Dixon, J. 164
Dodd, A.W. 120
Donaldson, L. 165, 166

Eakin, J. 113
Enthoven, A. 162
Evans, D. 86

Flint, C. 59–60
Frankena, W. 36
Franklin, B. 47–48
Freud, S. 66–67
Friedman, M. 71
Fukuyama, F. 108, 112, 134

Gastmans, C. 55
Gerkin, C. 10–11
Ghosal, S. 144, 157
Gibbs, R. 26
Gisèle 58–59
Graham, E. 11
Green, J. 56–57

Halligan, A. 166
Ham, C. 162
Hanson, P. 103
Hartrick, G. 55–56
Hauerwas, S. 45, 74
Herion, G. 105
Herman, S. 127–129
Heskett, J. 120
Hobson, R. 69–70
Hoy, W. 145
Hycner, R. 71

Janssens, L. 29
Jones, T. 179

Kainz, H. 35
Kant, I. 36–38
Kent, B. 72–73
Kenyon, M. 165
Kitson, A. 122
Kitzinger, S. 56, 57
Kohut, H. 70
Kotter, J. 120
Krajewsji, R 120, 139
Kramer, R. 144

Lane, C. 154–155
Lantz, J. 68
Le Grand, J. 162, 163
Lewicki, R. 142, 143
Lorenz, E. 149
Luhmann, N. 152–154
Lungren, I. 58

MacEachen, E. 113
MacIntyre, A. 17, 33–34, 37, 39, 47–50, 52
Mander, A. 115
Marcel, G. 12, 16, 17, 19, 23–31, 51, 79–82
May, R. 67–68
Maynard, A. 162
McCarthy, M. 139
McClendon, J. 33